Monographs on Endocrinology

Volume 18

Edited by

F. Gross, Heidelberg · M. M. Grumbach, San Francisco
A. Labhart, Zürich · M. B. Lipsett, Bethesda
T. Mann, Cambridge · L. T. Samuels (†), Salt Lake City
J. Zander, München

Inder J. Chopra

Triiodothyronines in Health and Disease

With a Contribution by V. Cody

With 76 Figures and 18 Tables

Springer-Verlag
Berlin Heidelberg New York 1981

Inder J. Chopra, M.D.

Professor of Medicine,
UCLA School of Medicine,
Center for the Health Sciences,
Los Angeles, CA 90024, U.S.A.

Vivian Cody, Ph.D.

Associate Research Scientist,
Medical Foundation of Buffalo, Inc.,
Research Laboratories,
Buffalo, NY 14203, U.S.A.

ISBN-13: 978-3-642-81550-8 e-ISBN-13: 978-3-642-81548-5
DOI: 10.1007/978-3-642-81548-5

Library of Congress Cataloging in Publication Data.
Chopra, Inder J 1939–. Triiodothyronines in health and disease.
(Monographs on endocrinology; v. 18) Bibliography: p. Includes index.
1. Triiodothyronine. 2. Thyroid hormones. I. Title.
[DNLM 1 Triiodothyronine. WI MO57 v. 18/WK 202 C 549 t]
QP572.T5C47 612'.44 80-27063

Typesetting: Oscar Brandstetter Druckerei KG, Wiesbaden

2125/3020–543210

Preface

The physiology and metabolism of thyroid hormones were areas of intense research investigation during the 1970s. Radioimmunoassays were applied to study the concentration of iodothyronines in biologic fluids. These techniques proved to be highly sensitive, specific, and reproducible as well as rapid. The availability of specific radioimmunoassays led to the detection of several iodothyronines in human biologic fluids, e.g., reverse triiodothyronine (rT_3), diiodothyronines, monoiodothyronines, and acetic acid derivatives of thyroxine (T_4) and T_3, which were previously either unknown or briefly considered but forgotten in the 1950s.

This monograph is intended for readers who desire an overview of thyroid hormone physiology as it was understood in 1979. It should be especially useful to trainees in endocrinology and individuals interested in potential research projects. The main focus has been on the studies conducted between 1969 and 1978, although other information has been reviewed to provide an overall working knowledge of the field. A list of over 500 references, although probably still incomplete, should lead a reader to at least a few important articles in each area relevant to thyroid hormone physiology.

The knowledge of several deiodinated derivatives as well as the production rates of thyroid hormones (T_4 and T_3) has raised several questions concerning the routes of metabolism of thyroid hormones along with the physiologic controls involved. In writing this book, I have examined the available information on various physiologic aspects of T_3 in health and their alteration in disease. In addition, key questions concerned with the understanding of thyroid hormone physiology have been reviewed; these include the following: (1) Is T_4 merely a prohormone for T_3 or is it also a hormone? (2) Is rT_3 merely a metabolic waste of T_4 or is it capable of biologic effects? (3) What is the nature of the processes of monodeiodination of T_4 to T_3 and to rT_3 and what are the factors that control these processes? (4) Why is serum T_3 low and rT_3 high in the fetus, in starvation, in systemic illness, and after the administration of some drugs? (5) Can the measurement of rT_3 in amniotic fluid serve as a prenatal index of thyroid function in man? (6) What are the routes of metabolism of T_3s, and are these routes altered in a characteristic fashion in some situations? (7) What is the relative potency of various circulating iodothyronines in the suppression of TSH?

The information covered in each chapter of the volume is as follows: Chapter 1 deals with the nomenclature, structure, and a history of the discovery of the triiodothyronines (T_3 and rT_3). Chapter 2 reviews serum binding of T_3s (T_3 and rT_3). Chapter 3, by Dr. Vivian Cody, reviews the molecular structure of T_3 and T_4, as determined by crystallographic studies. Dr. Cody analyzes the structure–activity relationship of thyroid hormones as it applies to serum binding as well as hormonal effects. Radioimmunoassay methodology for measurement of T_3s and the data on their concentration in biologic fluids during various clinical states is reviewed in Chap. 4. Chapter 5 discusses the data on metabolic clearance and production rates of T_3s, while information on the sources of T_3s is reviewed in Chap. 6. Chapters 7 and 8 discuss the metabolism of T_4 and T_3s in extrathyroidal tissues, and Chap. 9 is a brief overview of the biologic effects of iodothyronines.

Much of the data on the serum concentrations of iodothyronines is derived from the author's laboratory. The sections discussing the routes of iodothyronine metabolism, as reviewed here, should be considered gross estimates based on the available information. Sophisticated readers will no doubt appreciate the uncertainties and limitations of the analytic methods on which these estimates have been based.

Although emphasis has been placed on data from my research, I have reviewed studies from various other laboratories, especially in controversial situations. I believe these reviews to be fair. However, I beg understanding and kind consideration from those who may feel that an insufficient or misplaced emphasis has been associated with their contributions. If this has occurred, it reflects naivety and/or other limitations in the ability of the author.

Over the last 10 years, I have been extremely fortunate in my research to have benefited from the help and guidance of Dr. David H. Solomon, Professor and Chairman of the University of California, Los Angeles, Department of Medicine. He has been my mentor as well as a highly valued collaborator and colleague, and I am sorry that he was unable to join me in writing this monograph. Collaborative studies with Dr. Delbert Fisher of the Department of Pediatrics, University of California, Los Angeles, have also contributed invaluably to my work. I am grateful to Dr. Vivian Cody for contributing an excellent chapter on the molecular structure of thyroid hormones, which clearly enhances the scope of this monograph.

I am grateful to Ms. Guadalupe N. Chua Teco and Ms. Aimee Nguyen, as well as the other research associates and many fellows who have contributed so significantly to this study and to the overall knowledge of thyroid hormone physiology. I also thank Ms. Kim Harrell, Ms. Teresa Aguilar, and Ms. Kate Kavanaugh for their cooperation and excellent secretatial assistance. I am very appreciative of the skillful editorial assistance of Ms. Linda Olt.

The research of the author cited in this monograph was supported in part by USPHS grants AM16155 and AM17251 and the Research Career Development Award (K04 AM 70, 225) from the National Institutes of Health.

Los Angeles, December 1980 Inder J. Chopra

Contents

Chapter 1

Description, History, and Calorigenic Activity of Iodothyronines

Over the centuries, a sequence of events has led to the present knowledge of thyroid hormone physiology. Although not comprehensive, Table 1.1 provides an overview of the important milestones that have resulted in the present level of information and concepts.

Iodothyronine (initially termed "thyroidin") was apparently the first known physiologically active agent; it was discovered when extracted from the thyroid by Baumann in 1896. Kendall, in 1915, prepared a purer crystalline substance, which he named thyroxine. It was comprised by weight of 65% iodine and exhibited nearly all of the physiologic effects of other thyroid preparations then available. Harrington hydrogenated a solution of thyroxine in aqueous potassium hydroxide to obtain an iodine-free compound that he termed thyronine. His studies indicated that thyronine was an α-amino acid containing at least one phenolic group. He subsequently established the chemical structure of thyroxine and synthesized it as a 3,5,3′,5′-tetraiodothyronine (hence the abbreviation T_4) (Harrington 1926, 1933; Harrington and Barger 1927).

Figure 1.1 illustrates the structure of T_4 and other iodothyronines detected in biologic fluids. Iodothyronines are the only hormones known to be amino acids. Additionally, iodothyronines are the only naturally occurring hormones containing a diphenyl ether linkage. In the positions para to the ether oxygen, T_4 is substituted with a hydroxyl group in one ring and an alanyl side chain in the other (nonphenolic tyrosyl, α or inner) ring. The arrangement of iodine atoms 3,5,3′, and 5′ are depicted in Fig. 1.1. The aromatic rings are inclined at an angle of about 120° (Jorgensen 1964). The two aromatic rings can rotate about the ether linkage; this rotation may alter the important bond angle of ~120°. These and various other aspects of molecular structure and conformation of thyroid hormones are discussed in Chap. 3.

After the structure of T_4 became established, attempts were made to examine the relative importance of its various components, i.e., the iodine atoms, the diphenyl-ether arrangement, the side chain, and the hydroxyl group. Analogues were prepared and their effects were studied on the following: (1) basal metabolic rate (BMR) of thyroidectomized animals; (2) size of goiter in animals given iodine-deficient diets or goiterogens; and/or (3) metamorphosis of tadpoles.

It became apparent that any modification in the T_4 molecule with only a few exceptions (see below), yields compounds that are biologically much less active than the parent compound. Thus, the dextrorotatory form of T_4 has much less (~10%) activity compared with the naturally occurring levorotatory form. The finding that 3,5-diiodotyrosine (DIT) has negligible biologic activity suggests that the diphenyl-ether linkage is important to the biologic effects of T_4. However, iodine is also

Table 1.1. Some milestones in the present understanding of thyroid hormone physiology

Year	Author(s)	Observation(s)
1656	Wharton	Coined the term "the thyroid" or "oblong shield" to identify the gland. Its function: ? to beautify the neck, ? a "lubricant" of trachea.
1825	Parry	Identified heart failure with swelling in thyroid area.
1835	Graves	Described palpitation and enlargement of eyeballs as caused by associated thyroid swelling.
1840	Von Basedow	Described eye changes and infiltrative dermopathy in association with goiter.
1874	Gull	Described clinical features of thyroid deficiency.
1878	Ord	Found Gull's disease to be associated with atrophy of the thyroid gland, and called the disease "myxedema."
1883	Kocher	Described clinical features of thyroid deficiency after surgical thyroidectomy.
1883	Reverdin and Reverdin	
1884	Rehn	Performed subtotal thyroidectomy for treatment of hyperthyroidism.
1895	Magnus-Levy	First described the characteristic decrease in BMR in hypothyroidism and its increase in hyperthyroidism.
1896	Baumann	Discovered organic iodine in the thyroid, and named the iodine-containing material as thyroidin (later changed to iodothyronine).
1900	Gley and Bourcet	Identified organic iodine in the plasma.
1915	Kendall	Isolated thyroxine from bovine thyroid glands.
1922	Smith and Smith	Recognized anterior pituitary to be important in maintenance of thyroid function.
1926	Harrington	Devised chemical synthesis of thyroxine.
1931	Aron et al.	Found stimulation of thyrotropin secretion by hypothyroidism and its inhibition by excess of thyroid hormones.
1948	Taurog and Chaikoff	Identified T_4 as the thyroid hormone in circulation.
1949	Hoskins	Formulated the negative feedback hypothesis for pituitary thyroid axis emphasizing the homeostatic ("hormostat") nature of the system.
1952 – 1954	Gross and Pitt-Rivers	Identified triiodothyronine (T_3) in human thyroid and suggested that T_4 may be converted to more active T_3 as an important step in optimal action of thyroid hormones.
1951	Greer	Recognized importance of hypothalamus in release of TSH from the pituitary.
1952	Roche et al.	Identified T_3 in rat thyroid and reported its synthesis by iodinating 3,5-diiodothyronine (3,5-T_2).
1952	Gordon et al.	Demonstrated binding of T_4 in plasma to a protein migrating during zone electrophoresis on paper in the region of α-globulins.
1952	Robbins and Rall	Confirmed and extended this finding by showing that protein carrier of T_4 in serum migrates during paper electrophoresis in the region between α_1- and α_2-globulins. This protein has been called thyroxine-binding globulin (TBG).
1952	Larson et al.	
1952	Winzler and Notrica	
1956	Roche et al.	Identified 3,3′5′-triiodothyronine (rT_3) and 3,3′-diiodothyronine (3,3′-T_2) in the thyroid gland and/or plasma of the rat.
1958	Ingbar	Demonstrated binding of T_4 to thyroxine-binding prealbumin (TBPA) in serum.
1966	Schally et al.	Characterized TRH from porcine hypothalamus as containing three amino acids, histidine, glutamine, and proline.

Table 1.1 (continued)

Year	Author(s)	Observation(s)
1969 1969	Burgus et al. Shally et al.	Devised chemical synthesis of a tripeptide, L-pyroglutamyl-L-histidyl-L-proline amide which had the full biologic activity of TRH isolated from hypothalamus. TRH was thus the first hypothalamic hormone to be available in a synthetic form.
1970	Braverman et al.	Confirmed and reactivated the concept of conversion of T_4 to T_3 in extrahyroidal tissues.
1970 1971	Sterling et al. Pittman et al.	Provided data supporting Braverman et al. (1970) that peripheral conversion of T_4 to T_3 is an important source of T_3 in man. Similar information was also obtained in rats (Schwartz et al. 1971) and in sheep (Fisher et al. 1972).
1971	Chopra et al.	Suggested that thyroidal secretion probably contributes only a minor fraction of serum T_3 in man. (Chopra et al. 1971 a, Chopra and Solomon 1972)
1973	Surks et al.	Obtained data in T_4-treated hypothyroid patients which suggested that about 90% of T_3 in serum of normal man derives from extrathyroidal metabolism of T_4. These studies helped establish the information from other studies (see above) that peripheral metabolism of T_4 and not thyroidal secretion is the main source of T_3 in man.
1972	Larsen	Noted low serum T_3 and normal or high serum T_4 in the newborn cord blood. The basis for this intriguing finding was not apparent, however.
1972	Oppenheimer et al.	Described the presence of relatively specific binding sites for T_3 in the nuclei of rat tissues. This finding set the stage for important studies concerning the mechanism of action of thyroid hormones by this and other groups.
1973	Reichlin et al.	Noted low serum and tissue T_3 and normal T_4 in apparently euthyroid adults dying from nonthyroidal illnesses and suggested decreased peripheral conversion of T_4 to T_3 as the explanation for the finding.
1974 1974	Chopra et al. Carter et al.	Found low serum total and free T_3 and normal or high serum free T_4 in clinically euthyroid patients with a nonthyroidal illness and attributed low T_3 to reduced extrathyroidal conversion of T_4 to T_3. Carter et al. (1974) made similar observations independently.
1974	Chopra	Identified rT_3 in human serum and thyroglobulin; observed T_4 to be the major source of rT_3; observed a circumstance (fetal life) where serum T_3 is low and serum rT_3 is high.
1975 – 1976	Hesch et al. Visser et al. Chiraseveenprapund et al.	Demonstrated extrathyroidal conversion of T_4 to T_3 in vitro.
1975 1975	Vagenakis et al. Chopra et al. (a–d)	Found low serum T_3, high rT_3 and normal T_4 in healthy subjects undergoing complete fasting, in systemic illnesses and after administration of some drugs.
1976	Chopra	Suggested that thyroidal secretion contributes a small fraction of daily production of rT_3 in man and demonstrated that production rate of rT_3 is normal or high in nonthyroidal illness at a time when T_3 production is clearly reduced and T_4 production is normal or slightly low.
1977	Chopra	Presented data supporting the concept that conversion of T_4 to T_3 is enzymic in nature and demonstrated that other metabolites of T_4 (e.g., rT_3 and 3′, 5′–T_2) are potent inhibitors of conversion.

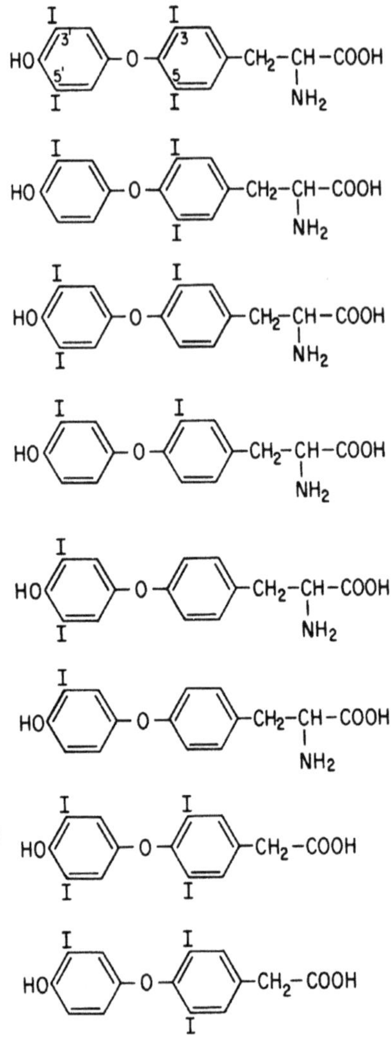

3,5,3',5'-Thyroxine (T4)

3,5,3'-Triiodothyronine (T3)

3,3',5'-Triiodothyronine (reverse T3, rT3, T'3)

3,3'-Diiodothyronine (3,3'-T2)

3',5'-Diiodothyronine (3',5'-T2)

3'-Monoiodothyronine (3'-T1)

3,5,3',5'-Tetraiodothyroacetic acid (Tetrac)

3,5,3'-Triiodothyroacetic acid (Triac)

Fig. 1.1. Structural formulas of iodothyronines and their analogues detectable in human blood. In addition to the compounds shown, 3,5-diiodothyronine (3,5-T_2) and 3-monoiodothyronine are also present in human circulation (unpublished data). 3,5-T_2 differs from 3',5'-T_2 in that the former has both iodine atoms in the inner ring instead of the outer ring. 3-T_1 has only one iodine atom, which is located in the inner ring. Pittman and Chambers (1969) have identified thyronine in rat urine. It is likely that this compound is also present in human circulation and urine as the ultimate deiodinated product of thyronines. (Chopra et al. 1978c)

important since thyronine, without iodine, has little or no activity. The substitution of iodine with other halogens (e.g., bromine, chlorine) markedly reduces the biologic effects of the molecule. Alterations in the side chain of T_4 cause a marked reduction in the activity of T_4. Thus, thyroxamine, which differs from T_4 only in that it lacks the carboxyl group in the side chain, has little thyromimetic activity (Gaddum 1930). Alteration in the phenolic hydroxyl group at the 4' position to methyl ether (CH_3O) reduces the biologic activity of the molecule to only about 5%

of that of T_4. Similarly, change from the oxygen group to a sulfur group for coupling of the benzene rings yields a compound that has only 10% of the activity of natural T_4 (Means 1954, Jorgensen 1964). It is clear, therefore, that all the components of natural T_4 have been devised to achieve biologically the most efficient compound.

There are a few exceptions to the last statement, however. Removal of an iodine atom from the outer ring of T_4 yields 3,5,3′-triiodothyronine (T_3), a compound that is two to four times more active than T_4. Similarly, if the iodine atom in the outer ring of T_3 is substituted by an isopropyl [$CH(CH_3)_2$] residue, the resulting compound (3,5-diiodo-3′-isopropyl thyronine) is two to three times more active than T_3. Interestingly, however, if isopropyl groups are substituted in place of iodine atoms in the outer ring of T_4, the resulting compound is inactive (Greenberg et al. 1963).

Like the discovery of T_4, observation of T_3 in the thyroid and in plasma has been a very important milestone in the present understanding of thyroid physiology. The discovery of T_3 depended on the availability of radioactive iodine (^{131}I) and chromatographic techniques for research studies. While analyzing by chromatography the components of hydrolysates of the thyroid glands of rats given ^{131}I Gross and coworkers (Gross et al. 1950; Gross and Leblond 1951; Gross and Pitt-Rivers 1952) observed the presence of an unknown compound, which was also an iodinated compound found in the plasma of these animals. Gross and Pitt-Rivers also found this unknown compound in the plasma of patients who had received ^{131}I for therapeutic purposes. Its chromatographic characteristics did not correspond with those of any of thyroxine analogues then available. This led Gross and Pitt-Rivers to synthesize 3,5,3′-T_3 by iodinating 3,5-diiodothyronine (3,5-T_2) and to study its characteristics. They found T_3 to behave just like the unknown compound in their sytems of chromatography. Subsequently, Gross and Pitt-Rivers (1952, 1953) were successful in isolating T_3 from the thyroid gland. At approximately the same time, Roche et al. (1952 a, b) also succeeded in synthesizing T_3 from 3,5-T_2 and in demonstrating its presence in thyroid glands of rats given ^{131}I.

The discovery of T_3 in the thyroid gland and in plasma was especially important because studies that followed showed this compound to be much more active than T_4. Furthermore, since the period between the time of administration and the peak metabolic effect was also much shorter in the case of T_3 than in that of T_4, it was speculated that T_3 may possibly be the principal hormone responsible for the peripheral tissue effects of the thyroid gland. This possibility was partially supported by the finding that T_3 is produced in various tissues (Kalant et al. 1955; Pitt-Rivers et al. 1955). Some in vitro studies also showed conversion of T_4 to T_3 by peripheral tissues (Albright et al. 1954). However, because other studies did not support this observation (Lassiter and Stanbury 1958,, interest in the subject was subdued and some 12 years passed before the concept became reactivated. The extrathyroidal conversion of T_4 to T_3 has now been demonstrated and confirmed; it actually has been one of the most active areas of thyroid-related investigation in recent years.

In addition to 3,5,3′-T_3, one other triiodothyronine, rT_3 (3,3′,5′-T_3, Fig. 1.1), has also been detected in biologic fluids. It is so called because of the location of three iodine atoms in this molecule is opposite of that in T_3. Thus, whereas T_3 has one iodine atom in the outer ring and two in the inner ring, rT_3 has two iodine atoms in the outer ring and one in the inner ring (Fig. 1.1). This difference in the arrangement of the iodine atoms in the iodothyronine molecule makes a marked differnce in its biologic activity. Thus, while T_3 is calorigenically two to four times as active as is T_4, rT_3 has less than 1% the activity of T_4 (Stasilli et al. 1959). Reverse T_3 has actually been shown to possess anti-T_4 effects. In pharmacologic doses, it reduces the metabolism stimulating effects of T_4 in hypothyroid patients (Barker et al. 1960). Pharmacologic doses have also been shown to reduce oxygen consumption in hyperthyroid patients (Benua et al. 1959). Interestingly, rT_3 has shown an ability to inhibit extrathyroidal conversion of T_4 to T_3 in vitro (Larson and Albright 1961; Chopra 1977). Whether or not the reduction in oxygen consumption observed after the administration of rT_3 to T_4-treated hypothyroid patients resulted from the T_4 to T_3 conversion-inhibiting effects of rT_3 is still a matter of speculation.

The presence of rT_3 was first shown in the thyroid gland of the rat in 1956 (Roche et al. 1956). However, the finding evoked a relatively limited interest, apparently because: (1) the substance did not prove to be active in calorigenesis (Stasilli et al. 1959) and (2) studies on the metabolism of radioactive rT_3 in man suggested that rT_3 may not exist naturally (Dunn and Stanbury 1958).

The studies of Surks and Oppenheimer (1971) stimulated interest in reexamining the possibility of the existence of rT_3 in the biologic fluids. These investigators proposed that iodine atoms from both the outer and the inner rings of T_4 are removed randomly at a similar rate resulting in the formation of T_3 when monodeiodination occurs first in the outer ring, or of rT_3 when monodeiodination occurs first in the inner ring. By this time, sufficient experience had been gathered in radioimmunoassay (RIA) studies of iodothyronines (Chopra et al. 1971 a, b, c; 1972a; Chopra 1971, 1972); it therefore seemed possible to obtain an antiserum against rT_3 that could differentiate rT_3 from T_3 or T_4 and other similar compounds. Studies verified this impression and using nonradioactive rT_3 prepared by Dr. R. I. Meltzer, (Warner Lambert Research Institutes, Morris Plains, New Jersey) and radioactive rT_3 prepared by Mr. B. J. Green and his associate Mr. Paul Shaddon, (Abbott Labs, North Chicago, Illinois) a highly specific RIA of rT_3 could be developed. Studies indicated not only that rT_3 is normally present in human serum and thyroglobulin but also that significant alterations do occur in its serum level in various thyroid diseases (Chopra 1974). Even more interesting was the observation that serum rT_3 is markedly elevated in some circumstances, e. g., shortly after birth (cord blood) and in nonthyroidal systemic illnesses, while in comparison with normal adult serum, serum T_3 is very low and serum T_4 is normal (Chopra 1974; Chopra et al. 1975 a, b, c). These findings have evoked much interest; several RIAs of rT_3 have become available and the basic data have been confirmed. Studies of the serum concentrations and production rates of rT_3, T_3, and T_4 indicate quite clearly that metabolism of T_4 to T_3 and to rT_3 is not a random process. The data actually suggest that pathway of conversion of T_4 to T_3 and to rT_3 are two parallel, and probably independent, processes, and that situations exist where one pathway (e. g., that of T_4 to T_3 conversion) is inhibited while the other (i. e., that of T_4 to rT_3 conversion) proceeds normally and may even be exaggerated.

Findings such as those just described suggest that peripheral tissues may be equipped with mechanisms that can modulate the extent to which T_4 should be converted to T_3 and rendered more active or converted to rT_3 and rendered inactive. In other words, it seems that thyroid hormone effects are controlled not merely through the now well-known, negative feedback system of hypothalamic–

hypophyseal–thyroid axis (Fig. 1.2) but also through mechanisms located in the extrathyroidal tissues determining the routes of T_4 metabolism.

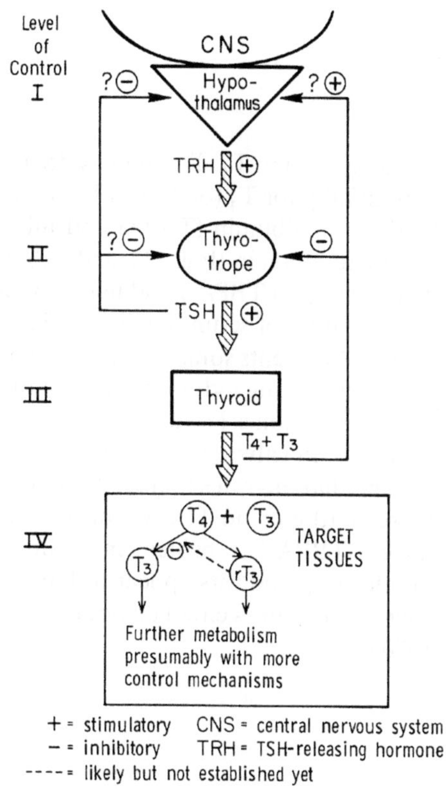

Fig. 1.2. Levels of regulation of the effects of thyroid hormones. It now seems likely that in addition to the well-known negative feedback system of hypothalamic–hypophyseal–thyroid axis, tissue effects of thyroid hormones are regulated by control mechanisms in the target tissues. These mechanisms apparently act by determining the amount of T_4 that is metabolized either to more active T_3 or to calorigenically inactive rT_3

Chapter 2

Transport of Iodothyronines

In human serum T_4, T_3, and rT_3 are bound to three proteins, which in the order of their affinity for T_4 (or T_3 or rT_3) are thyroxine binding globulin (TBG), thyroxine binding prealbumin (TBPA) and albumin. 3,3′-T_2, 3′,5′-T_2 and 3′-T_1 are bound mainly to albumin (Figs. 2.1 and 2.2) whereas tetraiodothyroacetic acid (TETRAC) binds avidly to TBPA in addition to albumin. There is at present little information on the nature of serum binding of 3,5-T_2, 3-T_1, or triiodothyroacetic acid (TRIAC). Table 2.1 presents some physical, chemical, and iodothyronine-binding characteristics of circulating iodothyronine-binding proteins in man. These proteins also bind thyroid hormones (T_4 and T_3) in the serum of subhuman primates and in horses. However, in calves, sheep, pigs, goats, dogs, and rabbits, albumin and TBG or a protein that migrates in the vicinity of TBG during electrophoresis are present, but there is little or no TBPA. On the other hand, pigeons, chickens, and kangaroos have a TBPA-like protein in addition to albumin, but they do not have TBG. Guinea pigs and rats appear to have neither TBG nor TBPA, and in these species thyroid hormones circulate bound to albumin only. (Farer et al. 1962; Refetoff et al. 1970.)

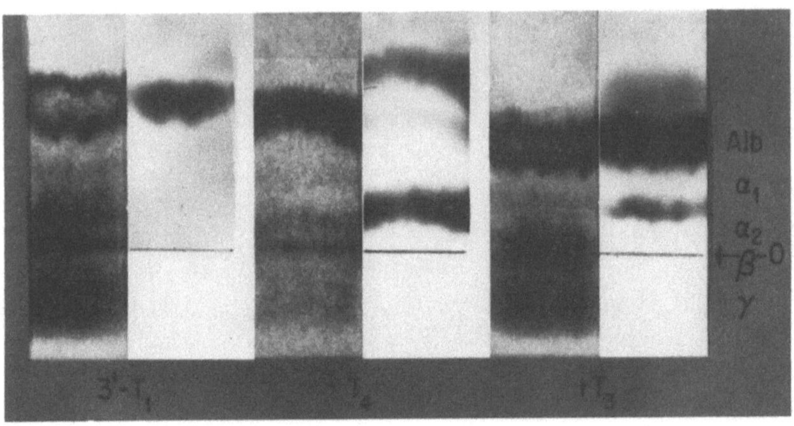

Fig. 2.1. Distribution of radioactive rT_3, T_4, and 3′-T_1 among proteins of normal human serum. Serum was enriched with radioiodinated (^{125}I) iodothyronines and subjected to reverse-flow paper electrophoresis in 0.2 *M* glycine acetate buffer, pH 9.0. Radioautograms for each iodothyronine are shown on the right of the strip stained for proteins with bromophenol blue. Alb = albumin; α_1 = alpha-1 globulin; α_2 = alpha-2 globulin, β = beta globulin; O = origin; γ = gamma globulin. In this electrophoresis system, TBPA migrates anodal to albumin, while TBG migrates in the interalpha globulin region

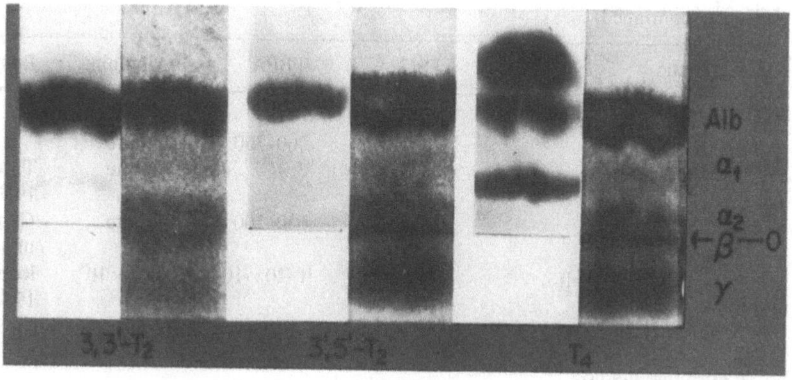

Fig. 2.2. Distribution of radioactive T_4, 3',5'-T_2, and 3,3'-T_2 among proteins of normal human serum. Serum was enriched with radioiodinated (^{125}I) iodothyronines and subjected to reverse–flow paper electrophoresis in 0.2 *M* glycine acetate buffer, pH 9.0. Radioautograms for each iodothyronine are shown to the left of the strip stained for proteins with bromophenol blue. Alb = albumin; α_1 = alpha-1 globulin, α_2 = alpha-2 globulin, β = beta globulin; O = origin; γ = gamma globulin

Table 2.1. Summary of recent estimates of various characteristic of circulating iodothyronine binding proteins in man

Characteristic	TBG	TBPA	Albumin	References
Serum concentration (mg/100ml)	2–4	25–30	4000–5000	Cavalieri et al. 1975 Levy et al. 1971
Volume of distribution (liters)	7.0	9.4	2.5	Cavalieri et al. 1975 Socolow et al. 1965
Half-life (days)	5.0	2.6	15–20	Takeda and Reeve 1963
Metabolic clearance rate (liters/day)	1.0	2.5	0.23	Oppenheimer et al. 1965a
Turnover rate (mg/day)	20	700–1000	10000	
Molecular weight	60000	70000	69000	
Sedimentation coefficient (SW20, $\times 10^{-13}$ s)	3.9	4.1	4.6	
Sialic acid content (%)	32	1.0	Low	Seal and Doe 1965
Tryptophan content (%)	1.4	3.2	Low	
Tyrosine content (%)	2.2	3.9		Oppenheimer et al. 1965 a and b
Binding to vitamin A (retinol binding protein)	–	+	–	
Distribution among serum proteins when tracer iodothyronine is added to normal serum and subjected to electrophoresis (%):				
T_4 (pH 7.4)	70	20	10	Davis et al. 1972
T_4 (pH 8.6)	60	30	10	
T_3 (pH 7.4)	78	9	13	
rT_3 (pH 9.0)	24	14	62	

Continued next page

Table 2.1 (continued)

Characteristic	TBG	TBPA	Albumin	References
Maximal binding capacity:				
MBC for T_4	20–25	200–300	Infinite	
MBC for T_3	15	?	Infinite	Thorson et al. 1969
MBC for rT_3	9–17	130–200	Infinite	Chopra, unpublished work
Km for T_4 (liters/mol)	$2–4 \times 10^{10}$	$1–20 \times 10^7$	$6–16 \times 10^5$	Robbins et al. 1974
Km for T_3 (liters/mol)	2×10^9	1×10^7	3×10^5	
Km for rT_3	?	?	?	
No. of hormone binding sites/mol:				
T_4	1	1	1	
T_3	1	1	1	
rT_3	?1	?1	?1	
Inhibition of T_4 (presumably T_3 as well) binding by barbital ions	No	Yes	No	Ingbar 1963
Inhibition of T_4 (or T_3) binding by salicylates, ANS	Yes	Yes	–	Wolff et al. 1961 Chopra 1971 Larsen 1972a Branch et al. 1971
Effect of administration of drugs on serum levels:				
Estrogen	Increase	Decrease	No significant change	
Androgen	Decrease	Increase	–	Braverman et al. 1968
Glucocorticoids	Decrease or no change	Increase	–	
Serum levels during nonthyroidal illness, protein-calorie malnutrition, and following major surgery	Decrease or no change	Decrease	Decrease or no change	Surks and Oppenheimer 1964 Bellabarba et al. 1968 Ingenbleek et al. 1972

A. Thyroxine-Binding Globulin

Thyroxine-binding globulin is the major iodothyronine-binding protein in the serum of humans. It binds T_4 most avidly (association constant approximately $10^{10}\ M^{-1}$); its affinity for T_3 and rT_3 is about one-third to one-tenth that for T_4 (Snyder et al. 1976; Chopra 1978a). Its characterization was initiated in 1952 by Gordon et al. who subjected normal plasma, containing tracer doses of radioactive T_4, to zone electrophoresis at pH 8.6 and observed that most of the radioactivity was located in the region of the α-globulins. This observation was soon confirmed and extended in several laboratories to show that TBG is an α-globulin that migrates between α_1- and α_2-globulins during electrophoresis (Robbins and Rall

1952; Winzler and Notrica 1952; Larson et al. 1952). Iodothyronines bound to the TBG are essentially nondialyzable and are not released by trichloroacetic acid or zinc hydroxide precipitation of serum, but are extractable by organic solvents such as ethanol and butanol. These characteristics of the TBG-iodothyronine interaction were usefully employed, initially in measurements of protein-bound iodine and more recently in measurements of serum T_4 (or T_3) by competitive binding radioassay in which diluted human serum was the source of TBG as the ligand-binding protein (Murphy and Pattee 1964, Sterling et al. 1969).

Thyroxine-binding globulin has now been purified to homogeneity by several groups (Seal and Doe 1965; Giorgio and Tabachnik 1968; Marshall and Pensky 1969; Sterling et al. 1971; Cavalieri et al. 1975; Refetoff et al. 1975). Its molecular weight has been estimated by four groups to vary in a close range of 54 000 to 63 000 (Seal and Doe 1965; Giorgio and Tabachnik 1968; Marshall and Pensky 1969; Refetoff et al. 1975), but was found to be lower (36 500) in the study of Sterling et al. (1971). Its sedimentation coefficient (SW) has been found to vary between 3.0 and 3.92×10^{-13} s. Initial studies suggested that the T_4 binding capacity of TBG is about 0.25–0.7 mol T_4/mol, but more recent studies suggest that earlier estimates may have been low because of the denaturation of TBG during purification and that TBG binds about 1 mol T_4 per mol. One mole of TBG also binds about 1 mol T_3 (presumably rT_3 as well) and 8-anilino-1-naphthalene sulfonic acid (ANS). Serum concentrations of TBG have been assessed by measurement of its maximal capacity for binding T_4 or by RIA or competitive ligand binding assay (CLBA). The maximal binding capacity of TBG in normal man approximates 25 μg/100 ml for T_4; this is higher than that of 16 μg/100 ml for T_3 and of 3 μg/100 ml for rT_3. The estimates of mean serum concentration of TBG measured by RIA and CLBA have varied between 2.2 and 3.6 mg/100 ml (Levy et al. 1971; Chopra et al. 1972b; Cavalieri et al. 1975). The serum TBG concentration is normal or slightly low in hyperthyroidism and normal or slightly high in hypothyroidism. However, serum TBG levels are clearly increased in pregnancy, during estrogen administration, and in an X-linked dominant inherited disorder of TBG synthesis. As measured by maximal T_4 binding capacity, increased TBG levels have also been reported in infectious hepatitis and acute intermittent porphyria. Serum TBG concentration is decreased during androgen administration, in some cases with hepatic cirrhosis, and in a genetic disorder of TBG synthesis (Levy et al. 1971; Chopra et al. 1972b; Refetoff and Selenkow 1968).

The kenetics of the matabolism of radioiodinated TBG have also been studied. Data indicate that the plasma half-life of TBG approximates 5 days, while the metabolic clearance rate and turnover rate are about 1.0 liter/day and 20 mg/day, respectively (Cavalieri et al. 1975).

Thyroxine-binding globulin is an acidic glycoprotein containing about 9 mol sialic (neuraminic) acid per mol protein (Seal and Doe 1965). Reduction in its sialic acid content by treatment with bacterial neuraminidase does not alter its binding capacity for T_4, but reduces its binding affinity and retards its electrophoretic mobility toward the anode. Studies comparing the metabolism of radioiodinated intact and desialylated (neuraminidase-treated) TBG indicate that desialylation causes a marked enhancement in the degradation of TBG and suggest that this may normally be the mode of TBG disposal. The liver seems to be an organ of key importance in the synthesis as well as in the metabolism of TBG. Thus, TBG synthesis can be demonstrated in vitro by isolated monkey hepatocytes (Glinoer et al. 1977), and hepatectomy of the rabbit causes a decrease in the clearance rate of radioiodinated intact as well as desialylated TBG (Refetoff et al. 1975). The property of liver plasma membranes to bind desialylated TBG has recently been employed in a displacement radioreceptor assay using rat plasma membranes and radioactive desialylated TBG (Van Lenten and Ashwell 1972; Marshall et al. 1978). The site of conversion of TBG to desialylated TBG is not known.

As measured by rat hepatocyte plasma membrane inhibition assay, the serum concentration of desialylated TBG approximates 75 μg/100 ml. It is elevated about fourfold in patients with alcoholic cirrhosis of the liver. High levels are also observed in patients suffering from malignancies with metastases in the liver (Marshall et al. 1978). Premchandra et al. (1970) have suggested the presence of abnormally high levels of desialylated TBG in obesity. However, this has not yet been verified by studies using newer techniques, e.g., hepatocyte membrane inhibition assay.

B. Thyroxine-Binding Prealbumin

Thyroxine-binding prealbumin is so called because during electrophoresis, it migrates toward the anode with a mobility greater than that of albumin. The binding of T_4 to TBPA was first shown by Ingbar in 1958 when he reported on the distribution of T_4-binding serum proteins during paper electrophoresis in tris-maleate buffer, pH 8.6. It has been generally considered that TBPA does not bind T_3. However, recent studies using polyacrylamide gel electrophoresis and ultrafiltration techniques do demonstrate modest binding of T_3 to TBPA (Davis et al. 1972; Larsen 1972a). In addition to T_4 and T_3, TBPA also binds rT_3 and 3,3′-diiodothyronine (3,3′T_2), 3′,5′-T_2, and 3′-T_1 are bound mainly to albumin and minimally, if at all, to TBPA or TBG (Figs. 2.1 and 2.2).

Thyroxine-binding prealbumin has been purified to homogeneity and characterized in detail by at least two groups (Oppenheimer et al. 1965a, b; Socolow et al. 1965). TBPA is a tryptophan-rich protein with a mol wt. 70000–73000. Raz and Goodman (1969) have shown that TBPA exists in human circulation as a protein–protein complex with vitamin A (retinol)-binding protein. They showed that the molecular weight of purified TBPA is about 50000 and that other estimates showing it to be about 70000 may have been caused by co-purification with TBPA of retinol binding protein which has a molecular weight of about 21000. It turns out that TBPA does not bind retinol-binding protein at the same site as T_4. TBPA binds one mol T_4 per mol protein. This information is not yet known for T_3 and rT_3 but is presumably similar to T_4. The mean maximal binding capacity of TBPA for T_4 has varied between 230 and 274 μg/100 ml in most studies (Balfour and Tunnicliffe 1960; Oppenheimer et al. 1966). It has not yet been reported for T_3. Preliminary studies in the author's laboratory suggest that the maximal binding capacity of TBPA for rT_3 approximates 140 μg/100 ml (range 137–195, $n=6$). Serum concentration of TBPA has been assessed by methods based on its maximal binding capacity for T_4 and by radial-immunodiffusion techniques; the mean values average about 25–30 mg/100 ml (Oppenheimer et al. 1966; Ingenbleek et al. 1972). Serum TBPA is increased during androgen treatment, while it is reduced in nonthyroidal illnesses and in protein–calorie malnutrition.

C. Free Thyroid Hormones

The concept of "free" thyroid hormones and physiologic purpose to iodothyronine-binding proteins may be explained as follows. As information on circulating thyroid hormones increased, it became apparent that the serum concentration of T_4 [measured as protein-bound iodine (PBI)] is increased in hyperthyroidism and decreased in hypothyroidism. However, it has also been found that serum T_4 is increased in pregnancy and in estrogen-treated subjects, often as much as in hyperthyroid patients, in the absence of clear evidence of hypermetabolism (Heinemann et al. 1948; Engstrom et al. 1952; Engstrom and Markardt 1954). Equally intriguing was the opposite finding of low PBI in euthyroid or questionably hypothyroid patients with the nephrotic syndrome; when treated with thyroid preparations, these patients, unlike typical hypothyroid patients, did not show clinical improvement or normalization of low PBI, high cholesterol and depressed BMR (Peters and Man 1948). While the abnormality in PBI could be explained on the basis of hormonally induced increases in TBG during pregnancy and the loss of TBG in urine with the nephrotic syndrome (Dowling et al. 1956; Robbins et al. 1957), discordance between serum thyroid hormone levels and the clinical picture raised several questions concerning the mechanism(s) by which circulating thyroid hormones enter into the cells to exert biologic effects and the physiologic purpose of thyroid hormone-binding proteins.

Data have not favored the possibility that T_4 enters the cell while bound to serum proteins. Early in vitro studies suggested that the transport of T_4 into tissues is a result of reversible equilibrium between extracellular and cellular T_4-binding proteins (Freinkel et al. 1957). A significant body of evidence has since been accumulated to indicate that physiologic effects of T_4 are caused by its small unbound, diffusible, or free fraction (Robbins and Rall 1957; Ingbar and Freinkel 1960). The normal free fraction of T_4 is about 0.03% and the normal concentration of free T_4 (which is derived by multiplying total T_4 by its free fraction) approximates 2–4 ng/100 ml. In comparison, the normal free fractions of T_3 and rT_3 are about 0.3% and 0.25%, respectively, whereas the concentration of free T_3 and rT_3 approximates 200–600 pg/100 ml and 60–160 pg/100 ml, respectively (Chopra et al. 1975d). The free fraction of iodothyronines is reduced when TBG is elevated and vice versa. However, the serum concentration of free iodothyronines remains normal and consistent with clinical euthyroidism. The concept that peripheral tissue effects of thyroid hormones are determined mainly by the concentration of free T_4 (and T_3) is also supported by the finding of relative constancy of free T_4 concentration in various species with widely differing serum T_4 and T_4-binding proteins. However, free T_4 concentration is lower in monkeys and higher in birds and fish than in man and other species (Refetoff et al. 1970).

Transport of thyroid hormones from the sites of production to those of action is clearly one important function of iodothyronine-binding proteins. Since extra-thyroidal metabolism of T_4 turns out to be quantitatively an even more important source of T_3 and rT_3 than thyroidal secretion, and since various body tissues differ markedly in their ability to generate T_3 from T_4 (Chopra 1977), it seems quite efficient to have an arrangement whereby T_3-binding proteins mobilize T_3 from "T_3-generating" tissues into the circulation for transport to all tissues of the body. Also, the presence of potent binding proteins in the serum may serve to reduce the distribution of iodothyronines to tissues with less "avid" binding sites, thereby making them more available to tissues equipped with avid binding sites for specific biologic effects and/or metabolism of iodothyronines. The concentration of TBG in serum is an important determinant of the rate of utilization of iodothyronines. Thus, the degradation rate (μg/day) of T_4 and T_3 is increased in hyperthyroid individuals but not in euthyroid subjects with a high TBG whose serum T_4 and T_3 may be in the range seen in hyperthyroid patients (Nicoloff et al. 1972).

Thyroid hormone-binding proteins in serum may also influence the biologic activity of iodothyronines. Thus, one reason for greater biologic activity of T_3 than T_4 in man and several other species may be the lower affinity of its binding to TBG thereby rendering it more available to tissues. This consideration is supported by studies indicating that T_4 and T_3 are biologically equipotent in species (e. g., some birds) which do not have TBG or TBG-like protein in their sera (Newcomer 1957; Tata and Shellabarger 1959; Adamson and Ingbar 1967). T_3 is, however, more potent than T_4, for example, in the rat, which also does not have TBG. As in man, however, rat serum binds T_4 much more avidly than T_3; free T_4 in the rat is about 0.08% compared with a free T_3 of about 0.8% (Chopra et al. 1978 b).

Chapter 3

Triiodothyronine: Molecular Structure and Biologic Function*

A. Introduction

The active component of the thyroid gland, T_4, was the first hormone to be isolated and to have its structure characterized. Moreover, because the thyroid hormones possess relatively simple structures (Fig. 3.1), scientists were led to believe that their mode of action would be easily understood. However, although thyroid hormones have been shown to elicit a multitude of biologic responses, the specific nature of their actions remains unclear. Thus, the impetus to synthesize and test many analogues stemmed from the attempt to define those features essential for T_4-like activity.

At the same time that a specific response for each of these hormones was being sought, a number of hypotheses had been proposed to relate the various structural features of these hormones to the expression of their biological effects. Among the many proposals suggested, the following were of key importance: (1) the unique role of iodine, for both its steric and electronic properties, (2) the diphenyl ether linkage in controlling conformation, (3) the 4′-hydroxyl for receptor binding, and (4) the side chain composition. The investigation of these hypotheses has been carried out utilizing such techniques as nuclear magnetic resonance (NMR) spectroscopy, theoretical molecular orbital (MO) energy calculations, and X-ray crystallography to elucidate structure–activity for the data of the thyroid hormones and their analogues.

It is generally accepted that a hormone must interact with some macromolecule to initiate a chain of events that results in an observed response. The presence of certain unique structural characteristics of thyroid hormones suggests that their

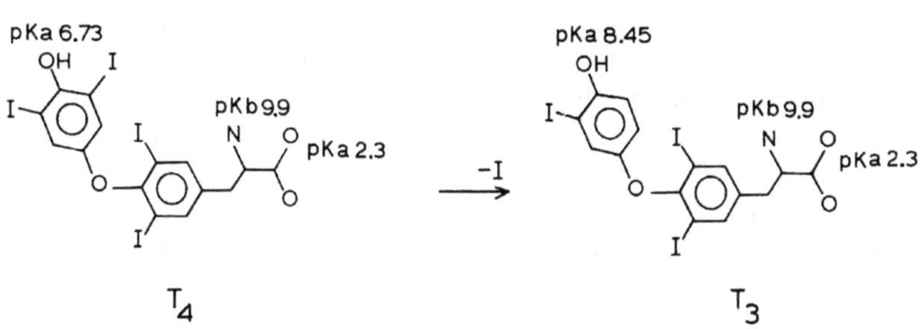

Fig. 3.1. Thyroid hormones: 3′,5′,3,5-tetraiodo-L-thyronine (T_4) and 3,5,3′-triiodo-L-thyronine (T_3)

* This chapter has been contributed by Dr. Vivian Cody.

action may involve a two step process: (1) binding at a specific site on the macromolecule, followed by (2) an interaction between some chemically reactive group on the hormone and a complementary component on the receptor, resulting in a chemical or conformational change in the latter. It is therefore, apparent that thyroid hormone function is dependent upon the three-dimensional structure of the hormone and its receptor.

X-Ray crystal structure determinations provide the most precise details possible of molecular composition, configuration, and conformation. Also, crystallographic techniques can be used to identify intermediates, metabolites, and their reaction products; delineate active hormone conformations; and develop mechanistic models for hormone action. Pharmacologic correlations can be made via comparison of molecular conformation with relative protein binding affinities. The delineation of patterns in conformational flexibility and the effects these conformational changes have on the selection of biologic action are the subjects of this review. Readers may refer to additional descriptions of structure–function relationships among thyroid hormones (Pittman and Pittmann 1974; Jorgensen 1976, 1978; Cody 1978 a).

B. Stereochemistry and Molecular Conformation

The thyronine nucleus constitutes the basic structural unit of thyroid hormones. By varying the degree of iodination, all presently known thyroid hormone structures can be derived (Fig. 3.2). Recent evidence indicates that all of these species are present in the thyroid gland. However, thyronine itself is inactive. It has an "outer" phenoxy ring and an "inner" alanine-bearing ring, and it can be described either as a diphenyl ether with an alanine side chain or as a tyrosine with a phenoxy side group. How the structural subunits of thyroid hormones are perceived may have some bearing on our understanding of thyroid hormone biosynthesis as well as their mode of action.

Early in the study of thyroid hormones it became evident that these substances possessed special stereochemical characteristics and that their three-dimensional features must be considered. Working with space-filling models, Jorgensen (1964) observed that the bulky groups ortho to the ether link caused the two ring systems to be nearly perpendicular and that these bulky groups hindered the rotation about the phenyl–ether bonds. These special stereochemical properties arise from the steric influence of the diortho iodines upon the diphenyl ether conformation. Minimal steric interaction between the 3,5-iodines and the 2′,6′-hydrogens is maintained when one ring is coplanar with, and the other perpendicular to, the plane of the two C–O ether bonds. This gives rise to two skewed conformations (Fig. 3.3). These studies led to the concept of preferred, if not somewhat rigid, orientations of the molecule.

An understanding of the exact three-dimensional make up of a molecule provides knowledge of its composition, constitution, configuration, and conformation. As illustrated in Fig. 3.4, composition defines the numbers and kinds of atoms that make up the molecule and is represented by its chemical formula. Constitution refers to the connectivity of the molecule and is illustrated by a line diagram showing which atoms are bonded to one another. Molecular configuration defines the

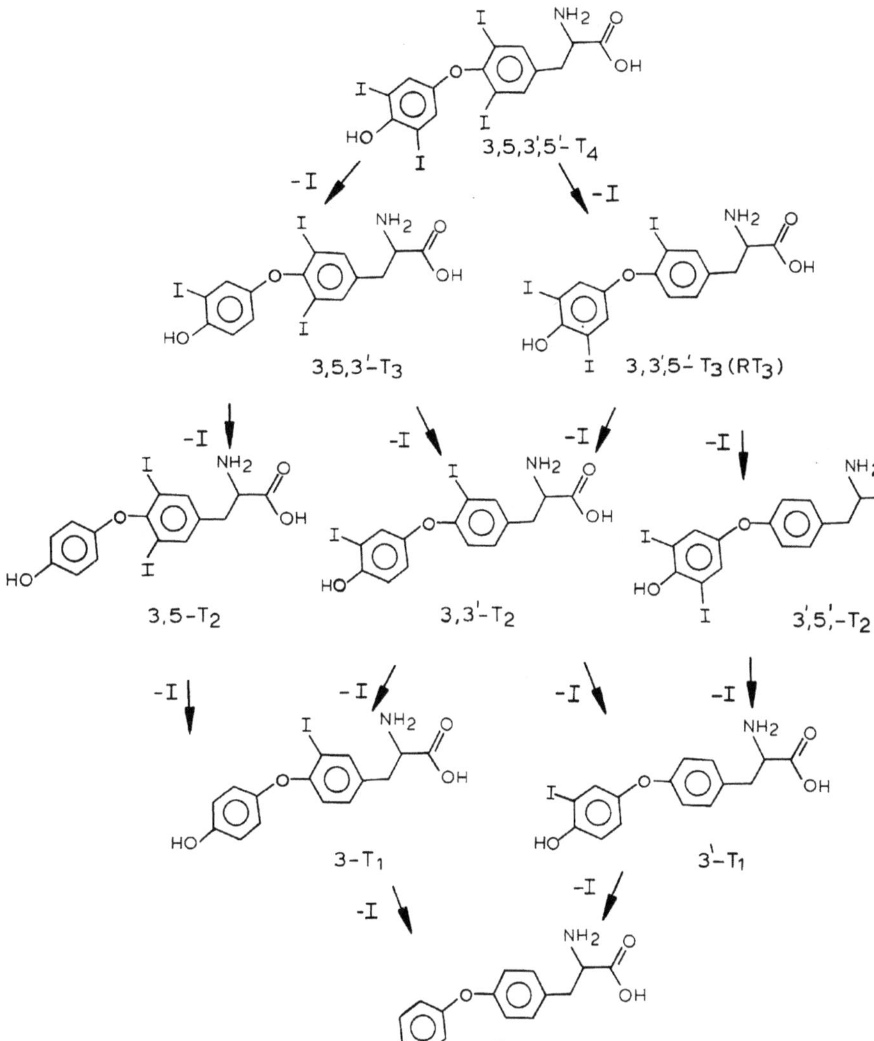

Fig. 3.2. Products of successive deiodination of thyroxine

chirality of all asymmetric centers in the molecule. Conformation refers to the total geometric distribution of disposition of the atoms in three dimensions.

For example, T_4, which is active, and 3,5-T_2, which possesses almost no activity, are distinguished by compositional and constitutional differences at the 3′ and 5′ positions. The functional dissimilarity between the L- and D-thyroid hormones stems from a configurational difference at the C8 α-carbon in the alanine chain. More subtle aspects of the functional dependence on structure are contained in the conformational features of the individual hormones. The rational development of functional analogues of thyroid hormones is dependent upon knowledge of these four components of thyroid structure.

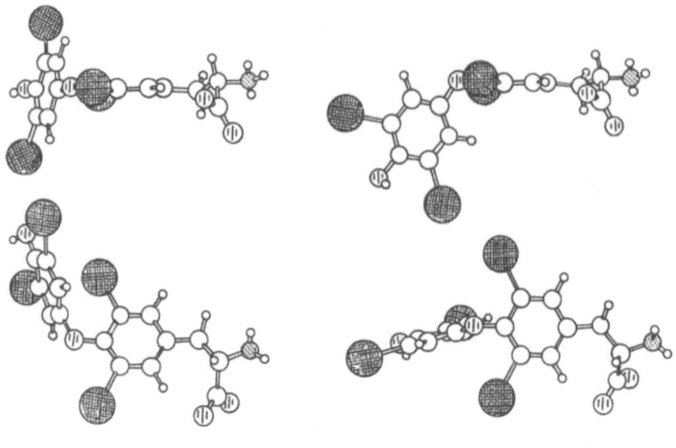

ANTI-SKEWED (φ/φ' = 0°/90°) SKEWED (φ/φ' = 90°/0°)

Fig. 3.3. Two examples of the skewed ($\varphi/\varphi'=90°/0°$) and antiskewed ($\varphi/\varphi'=0°/90°$) diphenyl ether conformation of T_4. In each case the molecule is viewed perpendicular and parallel to the inner ring plane

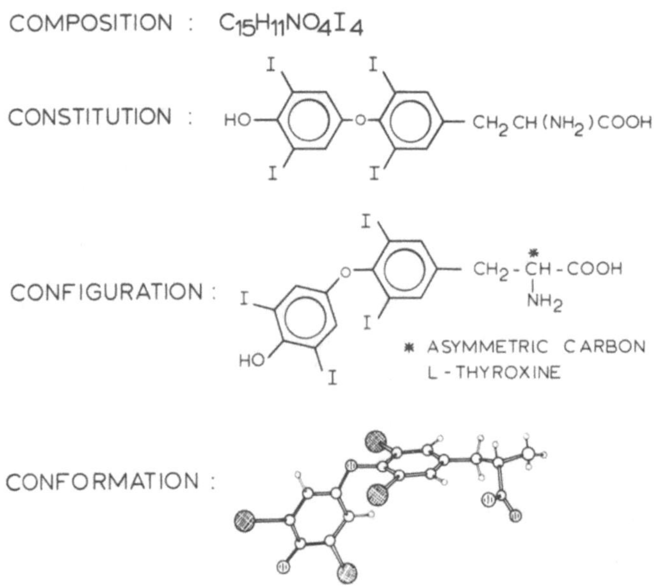

Fig. 3.4. Definition of molecular descriptors. (Cody 1978 a)

The first crystal structure analysis of a thyroid hormone nucleus was that of 3,5-diiodo-L-thyronine (T_2) (Cody et al. 1972). Since then, more than 20 structural determinations of thyroid hormones and their analogues have been reported. (Table 3.1, Fig. 3.5). A comprehensive analysis of these structural data provides a basis for the delineation of structure–function relationships from the interpretation of molecular conformation and intermolecular interactions.

The most important structural features brought to light by comparative analyses of all available crystallographic data on the thyroactive compounds (Cody 1976,

Table 3.1. Conformations of thyroactive structures[a]

Hormone	Structure	φ^a	φ'	χ^2	χ^1	ψ	References
TO01	3,5-diiodo-L-thyronine NMAE[b]	87°	21°	121°	−59°	17°	Cody et al. 1972
TO02	3,5,3′,5′-tetraiodothyroacetic acid methyl ester	−97	10	107	–	–	Cody, unpublished work
TO03	3,5,3′-triiodo-L-thyronine methyl ester	−104	32	121	−52	12	Cody 1975
TO04	3,5,3′-triiodothyroacetic acid NDEA[c]	92	−1	78	–	–	Cody et al. 1977b
TO05	3,5,3′-triiodo-L-thyronine	116	−21	76	−164	−7	Cody 1974
TO06	L-thyronine ethyl ester	114	−67	90	66	−7	Camerman and Camerman 1974b
TO07	3,5,3′-triiodo-L-thyronine HCl H_2O	90	−11	98	56	8	Camerman and Camerman 1974a
TO08	3,5,3′-triiodothyropropionic acid ethyl ester	−89	−10	46	–	–	Camerman and Camerman 1974
TO09	3,5,3′,5′-tetraiodo-L-thyronine HCl H_2O	105	−34	98	67	−9	Camerman and Camerman 1974a
TO10	3′-isopropyl-3,5-diiodo-L-thyronine HCl H_2O	98	−27	101	63	−2	Fawcett et al. 1976a
TO11	3,5-dibromothyroacetic acid NDEA[c]	98	−27	101	–	–	Cody et al. 1975
TO12	3,5-diiodothyropropionic acid	−100	4	101	–	–	Cody et al. 1977a
TO13	3,5,3′,5′-tetraiodothyroacetic acid NDEA[c]	−95	−4	129	–	–	Cody et al. 1977b
TO14	3,5,3′,5′-tetraiodothyroformic acid NDEA[c]	−103	8	–	–	–	Cody and Hazel 1976
TO15	2′,3′-dimethyl-3,5-diiodo-DL-thyronine HCl H_2O	85	23	74	41	−7	Fawcett et al. 1976b
TO16A1	3,5,3′,5′-tetraiodo-L-thyronine NDEA[c]	108	−30	152	−169	−40	Cody and Hazel 1977
TO16A2		−112	33	87	−160	49	
TO17	4′-methoxy-3,5,3′-triiodothyropropionic acid methyl ester	103	−21	99	–	–	Cody et al. 1978
TO18	4′-methoxy-3,5,3′-trimethyl-L-thyronine N-acetyl ethyl ester	−101	25	121	127	40	Cody 1978b
TO19	3,5,3′,5′-tetraiodothyropropionic acid NDEA[c]	−98	8	101	–	–	Cody, unpublished work
TO20	3,5,3′-triiodothyropropionic acid	−105	10	−16	–	–	Cody, unpublished work

[a] φ = C5–C4–O41–C1′, χ^2 = C2–C1–C7–C8, φ' = C4–O41–C1′–C6′, χ^1 = C1–C7–C8–N8, ψ = N8–C8–C9–O10

[b] NMAE = *N*-methylacetamide 1 : 1 complex

[c] NDEA = *N*-diethanolamine 1 : 1 complex

1978 a) concern the rotational flexibility of the five single bonds in the thyronine nucleus (Fig. 3.6), the restrictions upon the flexibility of these bonds, and the characteristic patterns of intermolecular interactions in these data. However, before

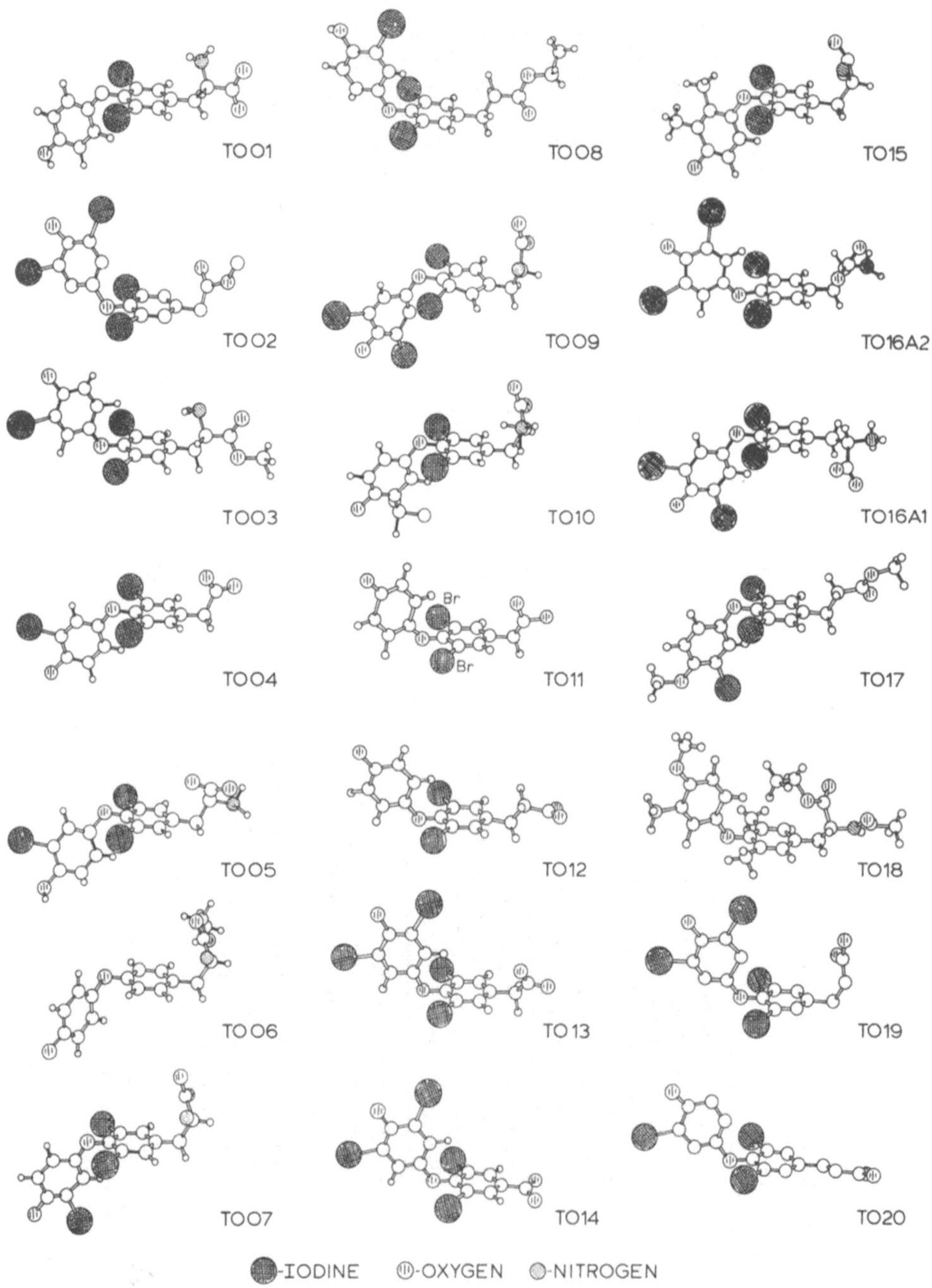

Fig. 3.5.
Observed solid state conformations of thyroid hormones. (See Table 3.1 for names and references.)

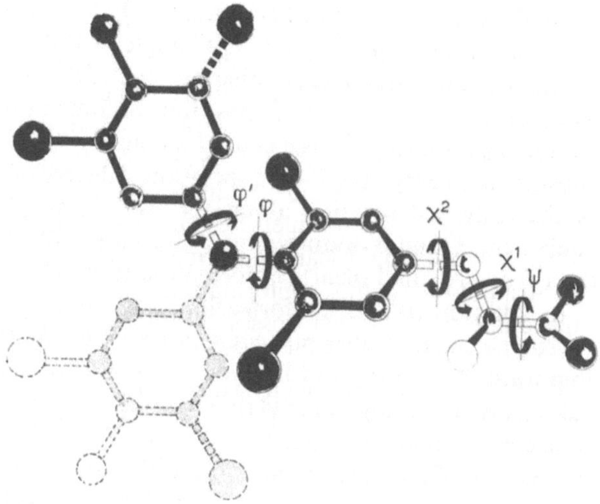

Fig. 3.6. Thyroxine with single bond rotations described. (Cody 1978 a)

conformational patterns can be described, the data must be labeled in a consistent manner.

Thyroxine is classified in *Chemical Abstracts* as an iodinated derivative of thyronine, whereas triiodothyronine is designated as a derivative of alanine. Consequently, a standard nomenclature giving a consistent numbering scheme of the thyroactive compounds which encompasses conformational as well as configurational features was adopted, as illustrated in Fig. 3.7. For convenience, a standard orientation was chosen in which the C8 α-carbon is positioned above the inner phenyl ring plane. The inner phenyl ring is numbered clockwise (when viewed from above), and the outer phenyl ring is numbered in such a manner that the C2′ atom is always distal to (away from) the inner ring.

Since the thyronine nucleus contains five single bonds, rotations about these bonds give rise to a number of conformations, many of which have been observed in the solid state. Consequently, the thyroid hormones are inherently more flexible than studies with space-filling models would suggest. This flexibility can be quantitatively described in terms of these rotations, as illustrated in Fig. 3.6. The flexibility of these molecules can also be described as having several basic aspects: (1) substituent influence, (2) side chain conformation, (3) diphenyl ether conformation, and (4) total conformation.

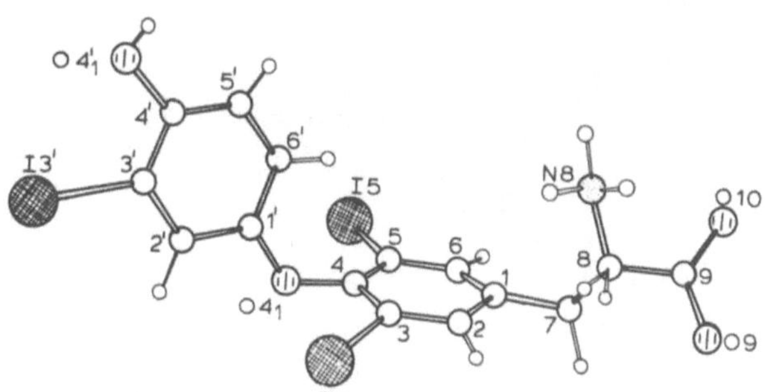

Fig. 3.7. Thyroid hormone numbering scheme and standard orientation. (Cody 1978 a)

On the basis of structural evidence (Cody 1978 a), it is found that the two phenyl ring systems are linked by a C-O-C angle of 120° and that the rings are disposed nearly perpendicular to each other because of the bulky ortho substituents. In such a conformation, the 3'- and 5'-positions become nonequivalent with respect to the alanine-bearing ring. In the case of a compound with only a single nonhydrogen substituent in either the 3'- or 5'-position, a degree of asymmetry is present. Because of the restricted rotation about the two diphenyl ether bonds, the chemically equivalent 3' and 5'-iodines are conformationally distinct, giving rise to a distal (away) or proximal (near) conformation (Fig. 3.8).

In addition to this conformational asymmetry of the outer phenyl ring, the thyronine nucleus also possesses other conformational properties that play an important role in thyroid hormone structure–function relationships. The alanine side chain on the inner phenyl ring has three single bonds that afford this part of the molecule a great potential for conformational flexibility (Fig. 3.6). The relative orientation of the inner phenyl ring with respect to the amino acid is described by the parameters shown in Fig. 3.9. Of all the accessible amino acid conformations, only a specific subset is predicted to have energetically preferred orientations (Ponnuswamy and Sasisekharan 1971), most of which have been observed structurally (Cody et al. 1973). Because of the specific conformational nature of the amino acid side chain, the overall conformation of the thyronine nucleus possesses special characteristics. As shown in Fig. 3.10, the observed preference for the C7–C8 bond to be perpendicular to the inner phenyl ring ($\chi^2 \simeq 90°$) gives rise to a situation in which both the alanine group and the outer phenyl ring lie either on the same side of the inner phenyl ring plane (cisoid) or on opposite sides of the inner ring plane (transoid).

As was pointed out by Jorgensen (1964), the bulky ortho substituents on the inner ring cause the two phenyl rings to adopt a nearly perpendicular conformation

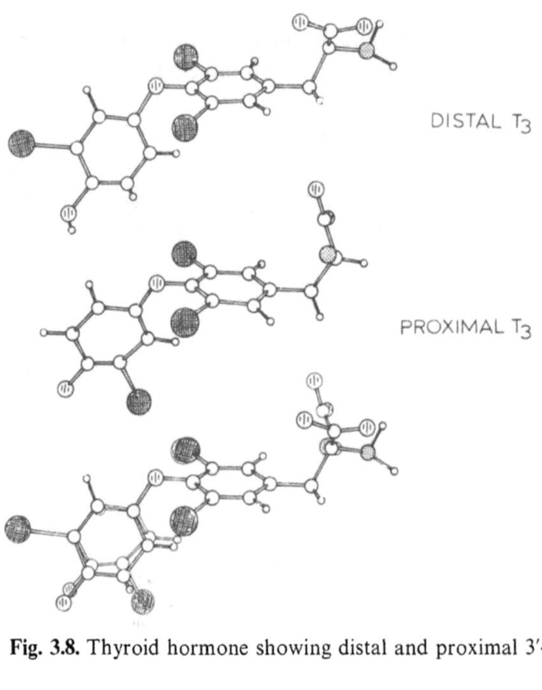

Fig. 3.8. Thyroid hormone showing distal and proximal 3'-iodine

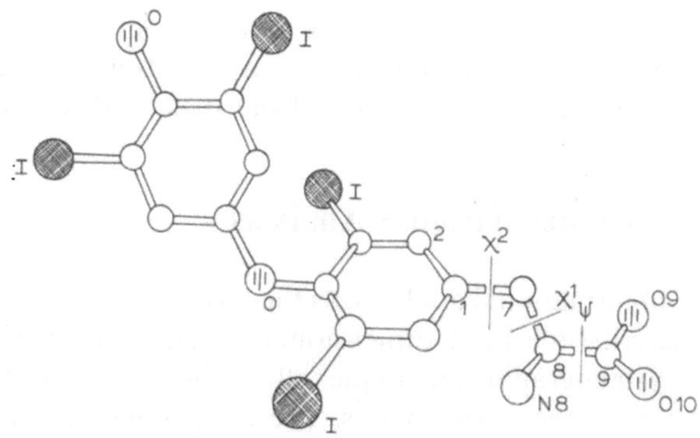

Fig. 3.9. Thyronine amino acid with conformational parameters defined

(skewed) about the ether bridge. This diphenyl ether conformation can be described by the rotations φ and φ' about the ether bonds shown in Fig. 3.6.

While the quantitative description of thyroid hormone conformation can be measured by the five rotational parameters[1] φ, φ', χ^2, χ^1, and ψ, (Fig. 3.6), it is an understanding of patterns in conformational flexibility and the effects these conformational changes have on the selectivity of biologic action that can provide

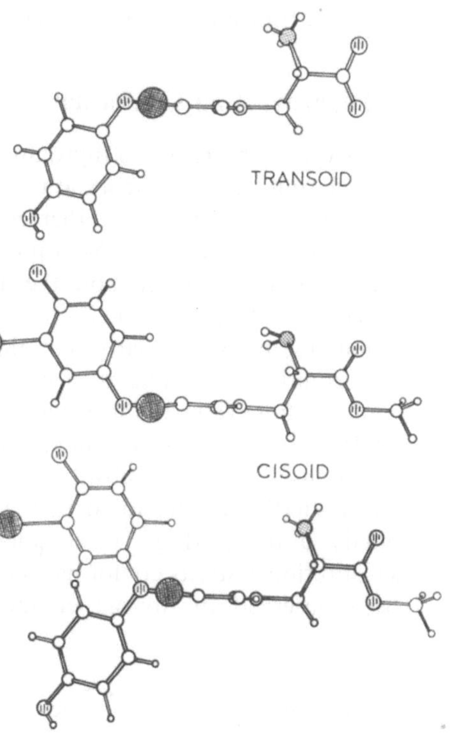

Fig. 3.10. Thyroid hormone illustrating transoid and cisoid overall conformation

1 These rotational parameters are defined by the following torsion angles: φ = C5-C4-041-C1′, φ' = C4-041-C1′-C6′; χ^2 = C2-C1-C7-C8, χ^1 = C1-C7-C8-N8, ψ = N8-C8-C9-010. A torsion angle A-B-C-D is positive if, when viewed down the B–C bond, the A–B bond will eclipse the C–D bond when rotated less than 180° in a clockwise direction (Klyne and Prelog 1960).

the necessary insight into the molecular level events that influence hormone action. The identification of sites of hormone action and the nature of protein receptors will lead to further elucidation of the structural requirements for hormone action.

C. Conformational Analysis

Conformational analysis, as the term implies, is the study of those parameters that describe the three-dimensional arrangement of the atoms in a molecule. X-Ray crystallographic techniques afford the means for the precise and accurate measurement of these parameters. Therefore, the systematic analysis of thyroid hormone structures by X-ray diffraction techniques provides not only the precise three-dimensional representation of these hormones, their metabolites, and their intermediates, but also a basis for the development of mechanistic models and, in conjunction with the other data, insight into drug design and receptor modeling.

Characteristic patterns of molecular conformation and geometry have been revealed by a systematic analysis of the structural parameters for the thyroid hormones and their analogues (Table 3.1). These data suggest that, in addition to delineating basic energy minimum conformations, there exist other, perhaps more subtle, correlations of molecular geometry with such features as pKa, ring substitution, side chain length, functional group orientation, long-range conformational transmission, and preferences in hydrogen bond directionality.

I. Diphenyl Ring Conformation

The oxygen bridge of the thyronine nucleus makes an angle of 120° with the two phenyl rings, and free rotation about the ether C–O bonds (Fig. 3.6) permits flexibility in the diphenyl ether conformation. However, the presence of bulky substituents at the 3- and 5-positions imposes steric restrictions to this flexibility, thus hindering rotation about the ether bonds. These special characteristics led to the concept of rigid thyroid hormone conformations with the phenyl rings adopting a mutually perpendicular orientation (Jorgensen 1964).

Currently many systems of nomenclature are used to describe diphenyl ether conformations (Higasi and Smyth 1960; Galasso et al. 1971; Van der Hiejden et al. 1975). From the measurement of dipole moments, four general conformations have been considered for unsubstituted diphenyl ethers: planar, perpendicular, skewed, and butterfly, as illustrated in Fig. 3.11. The rotations about the phenyl–ether bonds, φ and φ' (Fig. 3.6), describe these various conformations. Since diortho substitution restricts conformational freedom, only the skewed conformation has been observed in thyroid compounds. Table 3.2 demonstrates some of the

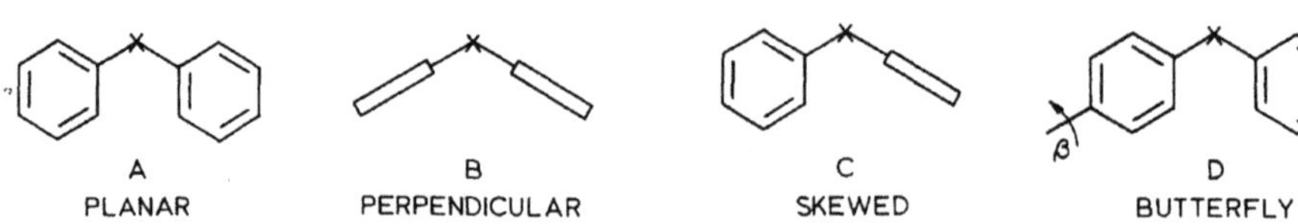

Fig. 3.11. Proposed conformations for unsubstituted diphenyl ether structures. The diphenyl ether parameters for these conformations are illustrated in Table 3.2. (Cody 1978 a)

Table 3.2. Diphenyl ether conformations

Structure 3,5-Diiodo-L-thyronine (TO01)	Conformation	φ	φ'	Comments
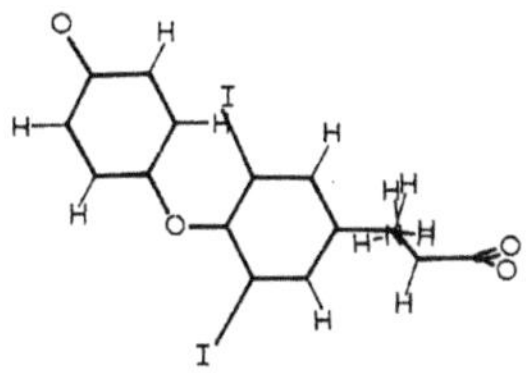	Planar	0°	0°	I–H 0.53 Å Unfavorable steric interactions, structure prohibited
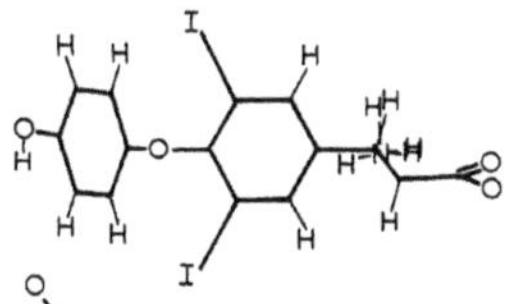	Perpendicular	90°	90°	I–H 2.29, 2.60 Å Steric interactions unfavorable, structure not observed
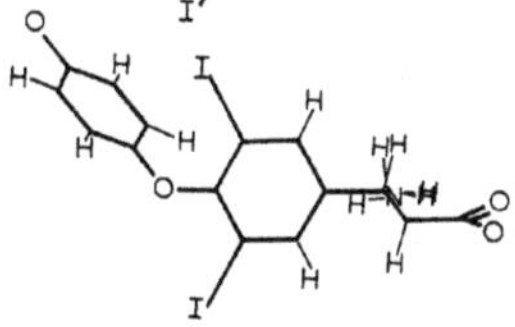	Butterfly	37°	37°	I–H 2.98 Å Steric interactions unfavorable, structure not observed
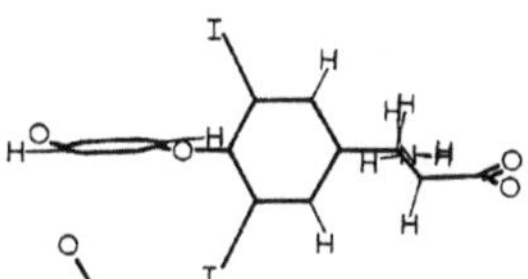	Skewed	90°	0°	I–H 4.76, 4.07 Å Favourable interactions TO01 observed with $\varphi = 87°$, $\varphi' = 21°$
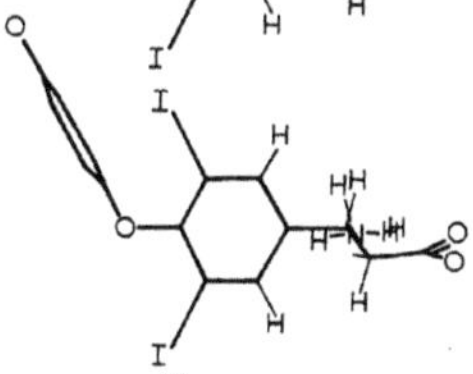	Antiskewed	0°	90°	I–H 3.42, 5.36 Å Favorable interactions but I–H outside range, structure not observed
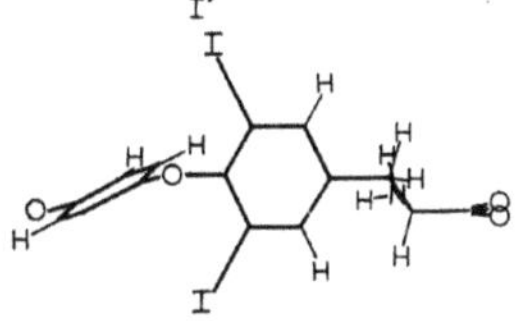	Twist-skewed transoid	108°	−28°	I–H 4.28, 5.33 Å Favorable interactions, but I–H outside observed range, structure in observed φ, φ' range
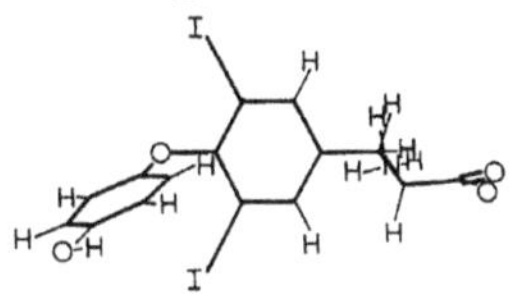	Twist-skewed cisoid	−108°	28°	I–H 3.86, 3.94 Å Favorable interactions, structure in observed φ, φ' range

interactions that characterize these ideal structures. As can be noted, severe steric repulsions are present between the iodine and the outer-ring hydrogens, precluding many of these conformations.

Because the diphenyl ether conformation is defined by torsion angles, the parameters φ and φ' are signed magnitudes and thus indicate the direction of angular deviation from the ideal skewed orientation, where φ and φ' are expected to be 90° and 0°, respectively (Cody 1975). As illustrated in Fig. 3.12, the torsion angle

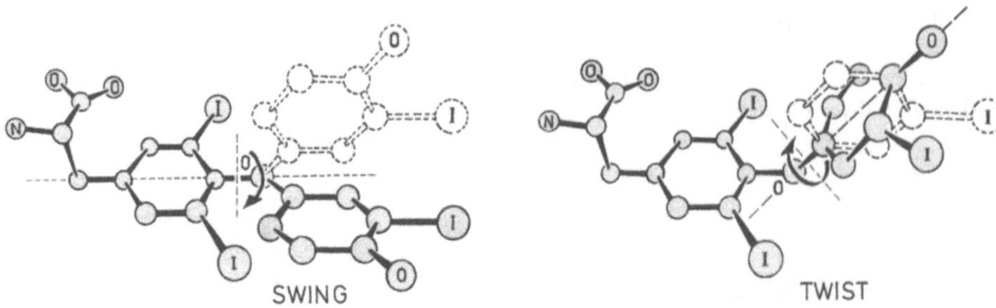

Fig. 3.12. Effects of φ (swing) and φ' (twist) rotations about ether linkage. (Cody 1978 a)

φ may also be interpreted as a "swing" about the C4–O41 axis while that of φ' describes a "twist" about the O41–C1′ axis.

Analysis of these parameters (Table 3.1) shows that the two motions are correlated (Table 3.3) and take place in a concerted manner, i.e., as the outer ring swings about its axis past the ideal skewed position, i.e., $\varphi > 90°$, there is a concurrent twist of the outer ring about its axis, i.e., $\varphi' < 0°$, in such a way that the steric repulsion between the inner ring iodines and the outer ring hydrogens is minimized. This minimum energy pathway is suggested by the linearity in the plot (Fig. 3.13) of the inner ring iodine distances to that of the proximal H6′ position. This linearity is not a function of the outer ring substituents, nor does it appear to depend on the absolute values of φ and φ'. This is demonstrated in Fig. 3.14 which shows the relatively constant H6′ position for divergent diphenyl ether confor-

Table 3.3. Diphenyl ether parameter correlations

Conformation	φ	φ'
Transoid	$< 90°$	$> 0°$
	$> 90°$	$< 0°$
Cisoid	$< -90°$	$< 0°$
	$> -90°$	$> 0°$

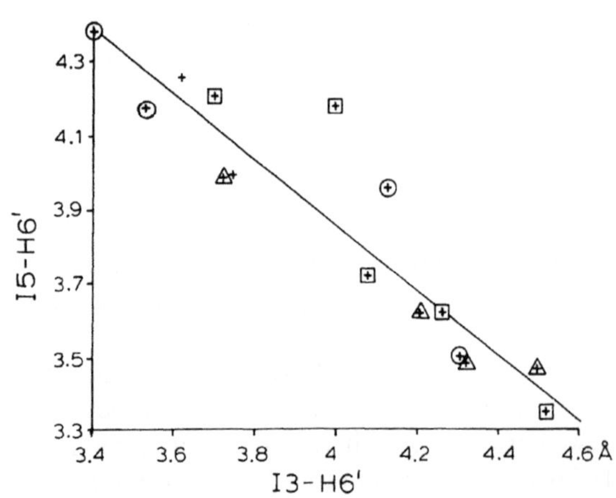

Fig. 3.13. Plot of I3-H6′ versus I5-H6′ distances for all thyroid hormone structures listed in Table 3.1. Those points enclosed by a circle are distal 3′-substituents, triangles are proximal 3′-substituents, and squares are tetra-substituted compounds. Points not enclosed are 3,5-diiodothyronines

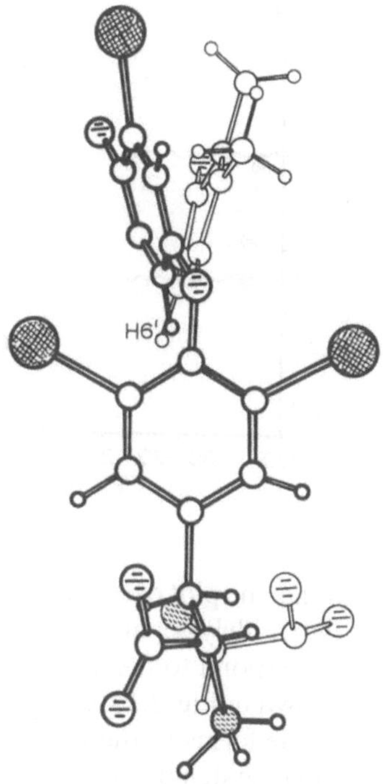

Fig. 3.14. Superimposition of TO05 (*dark*) with TO15 (*light*) showing the constant H6′ position for divergent diphenyl ether conformations (Table 3.1)

mations. A similar correlation exists for motions involving $\varphi < -90°$ and $\varphi' > 0°$. In this data base there is only one exception (TO13) to the relationships shown in Table 3.3; however, these correlations may not necessarily hold for other diphenyl ether structures (Cody 1975).

In general, diphenyl ether conformations have been reported in terms of the dihedral angles which are made by the ring planes and the plane of the central ether link, C4-O41-C1′. As can be seen by the comparison of Figs. 3.15 and 3.16 the torsion angles φ and φ' are the more informative parameters (Weeks et al. 1974). The plot of the dihedral angles (Fig. 3.15) shows a general scatter near the skewed conformation, but no correlation between parameters is observed. On the other

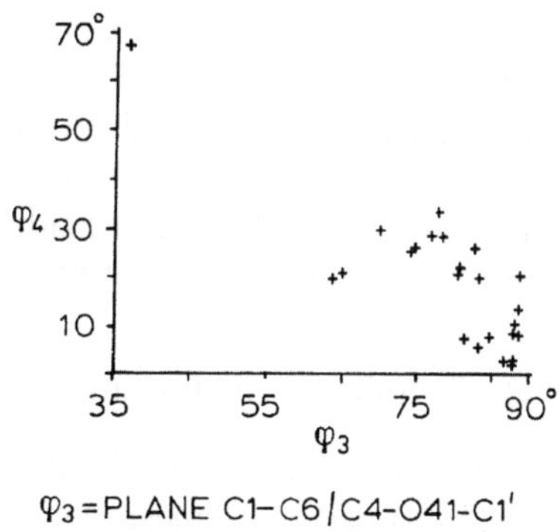

Fig. 3.15. A plot of the dihedral angles made by the plane of each phenyl ring and the plane C4-O41-C1′, respectively for all thyroid structures listed in Table 3.1

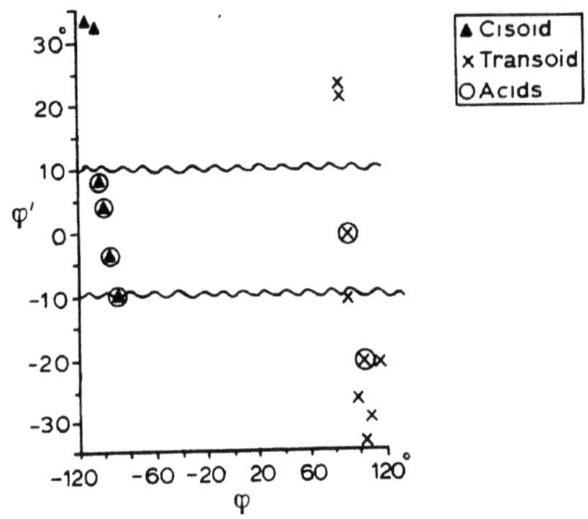

Fig. 3.16. A plot of the torsion angles φ (C5-C4-O41-C1') and φ' (C4-O41-C1'-C6') for all thyroactive compounds listed in Table 3.1. Wavy line separates $\varphi = 90°$ $\pm 10°$. (Cody 1978a)

hand, the plot of φ and φ' (Fig. 3.16) shows a discontinuity with the data falling into two widely separated groups. Upon inspection, these two groups are found to correspond to the cisoid ($\varphi \simeq -90°$) and transoid ($\varphi' \simeq 90°$) overall conformation shown in Fig. 3.10. Crystallographic studies alone brought to light the existence of stable forms of these remarkably different conformational isomers. Although the biologic significance of these conformers is not known, they are observed with equal frequency (Table 3.1).

Further analysis of the distributions seen in Fig. 3.16 shows other, more subtle, correlations. Those parameters of the deamino acid structures (thyroformic, acetic, propionic) are circled. With only one exception (TO17), these values fall within a 10° range of the skewed ($\varphi = \pm 90°$, $\varphi' = 0°$) conformation. Thus, it appears that the absence of the α-amino nitrogen, rather than its presence, influences this conformation (Cody et al. 1977b). The remaining amino acid structures are then paired on either side of this skewed range and, with few exceptions, fall into $\pm\varphi'$ groups for the cisoid and transoid sets, respectively. The average amino acid conformation can be described as "twist-skewed" with an average value of $\varphi = |108°|$, $\varphi' = |28°|$. These observations suggest that there are at least four variants of this conformation: transoid and cisoid skewed, and transoid and cisoid twist-skewed. The major difference between the skewed and the twist-skewed conformers (Fig. 3.17) is in the disposition of 4'-OH group or the side chain, depending on what part of the structure is held fixed. Depending on receptor-site binding requirements for the hydroxyl group relative to the stereochemistrv of the rest of the hormone, this difference may be linked to differences in binding affinities and hormone action. Furthermore, when the crystal structures of thyroid-binding proteins are determined, these data on the substrate conformational flexibility will be vital for the accurate interpretation of molecular details at the active site.

II. 3'-Substituent Orientation – Distal or Proximal

In the study of structural requirements for maximal thyromimetic activity, one of the most pertinent questions concerns the preferred conformation of the hormone T_3. Because of the conformational asymmetry inherent in the outer phenyl ring, it

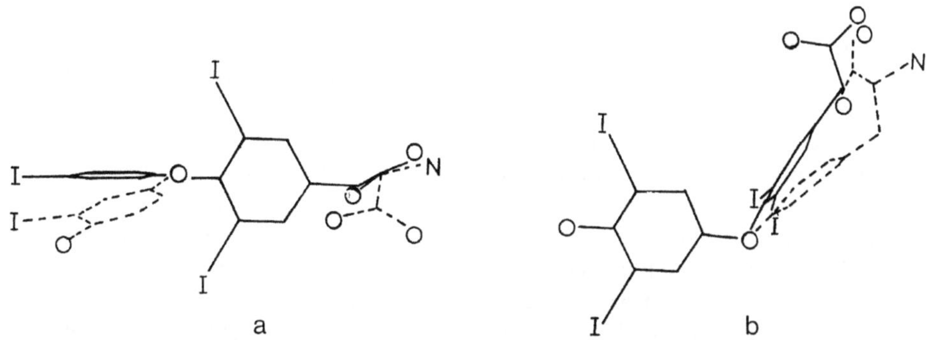

Fig. 3.17 a, b. A superimposition of TO04 (*solid lines*, Table 3.1) and TO05 (*dotted lines*) illustrating the differences between a skewed and twist-skewed conformation. **a** Overlap of inner ring as common structural feature; **b** The outer phenyl ring. (Cody 1978 a)

had been uncertain whether the preferred orientation of the 3′-iodine was distal or proximal (Fig. 3.8).

The conformational requirements for activity and protein binding were investigated with 2′,3′-dimethyl-3,5-diiodothyronine as the model for the distal conformer of T_3 and 2′,5′-dimethyl-3,5-diiodothyronine as the proximal model (Fig. 3.18) (Zenker and Jorgensen 1959; Jorgensen et al. 1962; Jorgensen 1964). These studies showed that the distal analogue is hormonally active, having 50% as much goiter-suppressing activity as T_4 and 13% as much calorigenic effect as T_3 (Jorgensen et al. 1962). The proximal analogue shows only 1%–2% as much activity as the distal analogue in these tests. Similar results were obtained in experiments using pure TBG or whole serum (Schussler 1972; Goldfine et al. 1976), indicating that the requirements for serum protein binding are the same as that required for hormone activity. Binding studies of T_3 analogues to nuclear receptor proteins also indicate a preference for a distally oriented 3′-substituent for maximal activity (Koerner et al. 1975).

Steric interactions of the inner ring iodines (Fig. 3.3) suggest a perpendicular arrangement of the phenyl rings "locked in" by a considerable barrier to internal rotation about the ether bridge. On the other hand, molecular orbital energy

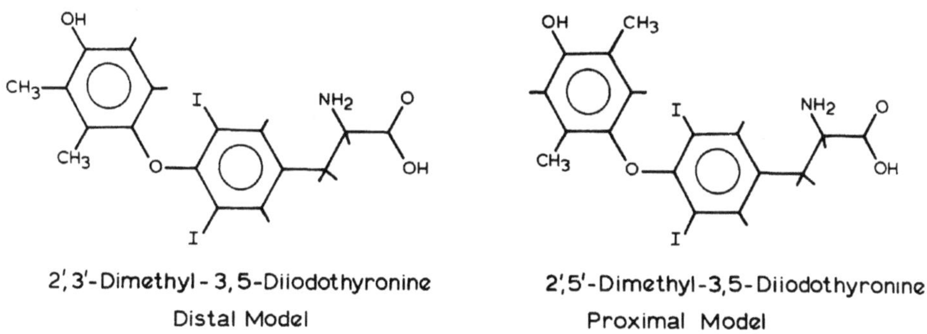

Fig. 3.18. Rigid model compounds used to test active conformation of T_3

calculations by Kollman et al. (1973) show a small energy barrier to rotation, although Kier and Hoyland (1970) suggest a considerable barrier to internal rotation. This barrier would then prevent easy conversion from one conformer to the other.

X-Ray crystallographic results obtained from the structures listed in Table 3.1 did much to resolve some of the ambiguities concerning conformational preferences of these hormones. Crystallographic determinations of trisubstituted compounds (Table 3.4, Fig. 3.19) not only verified the stability of both the distal and proximal forms of T_3, but also provided evidence that the relative stability of these conformers is sensitive to solvent and pH changes. It is observed that all of the 3′-iodo distal structures (TO03, TO04, TO05, TO20) (Table 3.1) were grown from neutral solutions, while the proximal 3′-iodostructures (TO07, TO08, TO17) (Table 3.1),

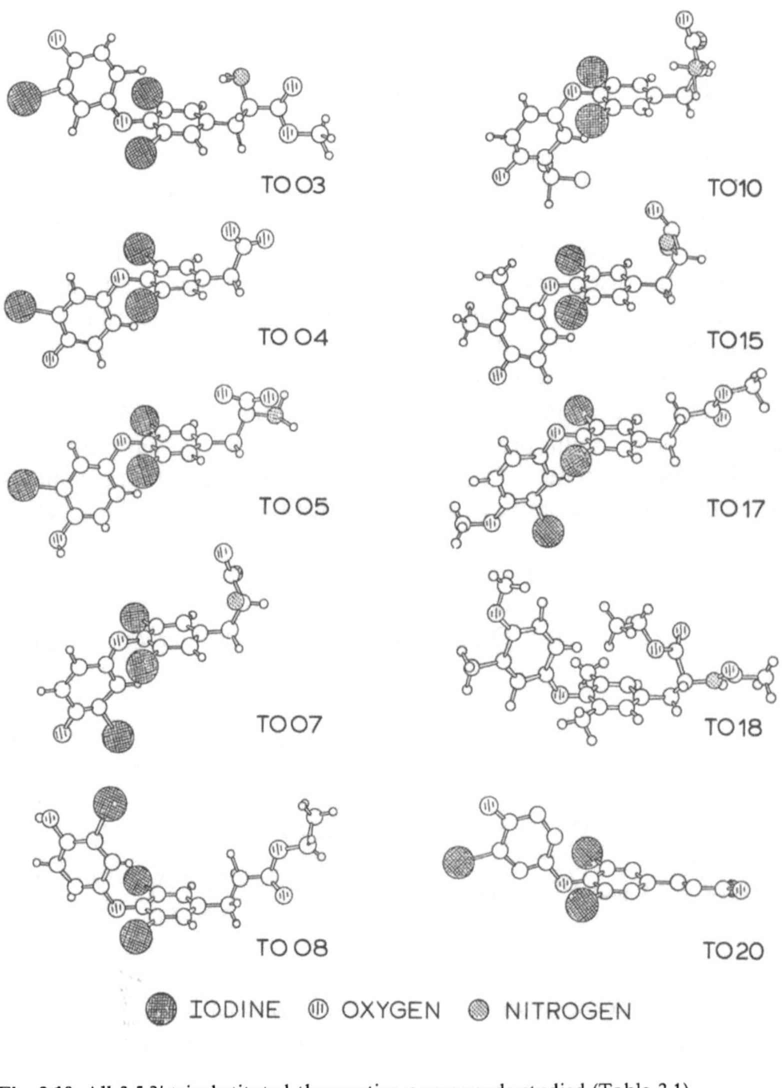

Fig. 3.19. All 3,5,3′-trisubstituted thyroactive compounds studied (Table 3.1)

Table 3.4. Conformation of 3,5,3′-trisubstituted thyronines

Structure		3′-Orientation	Overall conformation	Diphenyl ether conformation
TO03[a]	3,5,3′-Triiodo-L-thyronine methyl ester	Distal	Cisoid	Twist-skewed
TO04	3,5,3′-Triiodothyroacetic acid NDEA	Distal	Transoid	Skewed
TO05	3,5,3′-Triiodo-L-thyronine	Distal	Transoid	Twist-skewed
TO07	3,5,3′-Triiodo-L-thyronine HCl H_2O	Proximal	Transoid	Twist-skewed
TO08	3,5,3′-Triiodothyropropionic acid ethyl ester	Proximal	Cisoid	Skewed
TO10	3′-Isopropyl-3,5-diiodo-L-thyronine HCl H_2O	Proximal	Transoid	Twist-skewed
TO15	2′,3′-Dimethyl-3,5-diiodo-DL-thyronine HCl H_2O	Distal	Transoid	Twist-skewed
TO17	4′-Methoxy-3,5,3′-triiodothyropropionic acid methyl ester	Proximal	Transoid	Twist-skewed
TO18	4′-Methoxy-3,5,3′-trimethyl-L-thyronine N-acetyl ethyl ester	Distal	Cisoid	Twist-skewed
TO20	3,5,3′-Triiodothyropropionic acid	Distal	Cisoid	Twist-skewed

[a] These numbers refer to the listing in Table 3.1 and Fig. 3.5. See Figs. 3.8 and 3.17 for definitions of confirmations.

with one exception (TO17), were grown from acid solutions. The one proximal conformer grown from neutral solutions is also the only example of a 3′-iodo, 4′-methoxy analogue. These data suggest a pH sensitive equilibrium, which, at physiologic pH 7.4, favors the distal conformer. Thus, the methoxy compound, lacking a free 4′-OH, does not show this sensitivity. The crystallographic data indicate that these two conformers are stable isomers and readily accessible in solution.

The stability of the distal/proximal equilibrium was studied in solution using NMR techniques and the results are in agreement with these crystallographic studies showing ready accessibility to either conformer. Using model compounds, Emmett and Pepper (1975) determined a distal/proximal ratio of 0.56 in favor of a distal conformer at room temperature. They also studied the effects of temperature on this equilibrium and concluded, in agreement with other calculated values, that the barrier to rotation around the ether oxygen was small. This ease of rotation in solution explains why the early NMR studies of T_3 by Lehmann and Jorgensen (1965) failed to show two stable conformers.

Another attempt to observe either a distal or a proximal 3′-iodo conformation in solution was made in the NMR study of 3,5,3′-triiodothyropropionic acid ethyl ester (Camerman et al. 1975). However, these data led to conflicting results. The NMR spectrum of 3,5,3′-triiodothyropropionic acid in HCl–ethanol solutions was originally interpreted as a 3 : 1 mixture of proximal (major) and distal (minor) 3′-iodo conformations. Since there was no coalescence of peaks on heating, a large rotational barrier (>20 Cal) was computed. However, a reinvestigation of these data (Mazzocchi et al. 1976) showed the spectrum to be mixture of triiodothyropropionic acid and its ethyl ester.

In order to determine whether or not solid state conformations could be discerned in solution, further NMR studies of T_3 using lanthanide shift reagents were investigated (Cody et al. 1974). The spectrum of T_3 was examined in dimethylsulfoxide under anhydrous conditions in the presence and the absence of calcium and the lanthanide probes gadolinium, lanthanum, and europium. Using the crystallographic conformation of T_3 as a starting model, a solution conformation of T_3 was computed which satisfied the metal-proton distances obtained from the lanthanide-induced NMR shift data (Fig. 3.20). These preliminary results are consistent with a distal-cisoid model.

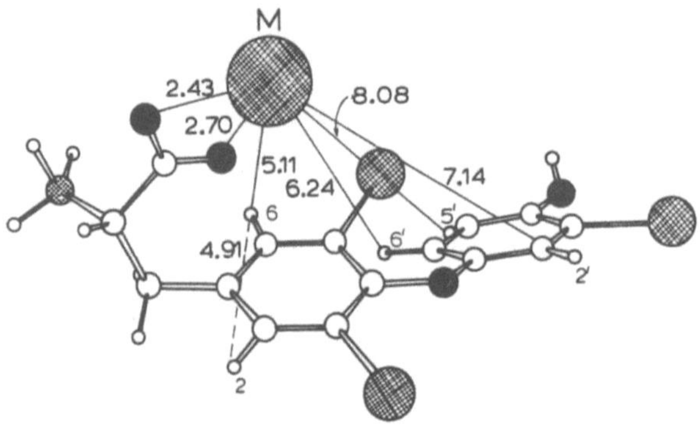

Fig. 3.20. Solution conformation model of T_3 based on NMR lanthanide shift data. Distances are the metal–proton distances calculated from NMR data; M, metal ion. (Cody 1978 a)

III. Side Chain Orientation

From a systematic analysis of 48 crystal structures containing aromatic amino acids (Cody et al. 1973), it was shown that these molecules adopt three basic energy minimum conformations. These conformations are described by the rotational parameters χ^1, χ^2, and ψ (Fig. 3.9) which delineate the amino acid backbone. This study also showed correlations among these paramenters for any particular group of χ^1. In the thyronine nucleus, χ^2 and χ^1 control the overall hormone conformation and therefore have a great potential to influence biologic activity.

The parameter χ^2 (C2-C1-C7-C8) in aromatic amino acids has an energy minimum conformation of approximately 90° (Ponnuswamy and Sasisekharan 1971). The χ^2 values from Table 3.1 range from 46°–152° and have an average value of 100°. This average is 103° for amino acid structures and 95° for deamino acids. However, it is this characteristic property that permits a distinction between cisoid and transoid conformations (Fig. 3.10).

Rotation about the C7–C8 bond, described by the torsion angle χ^1 (C1-C7-C8-N8), has the greatest influence on the side chain orientation. This parameter has three energy minima: ~60°, 180°, and −60°, all of which have been observed in thyroactive structures. As seen in Fig. 3.21, a value of $\chi^1 = 60°$ places the two functional groups in a folded position pointing back toward the inner phenyl ring, and it is considered the least favorable of the three energy minima. This conformation has been observed in those crystal structures (Table 3.1) that were crystallized from acid solutions containing HCl and H_2O in the lattice. This conformation is often found in amino acid structures that chelate metals (Cody et al. 1973). For those structures with χ^1 near 60°, the values of χ^2 and ψ tend to lie closest to their energy minima of 90° and 0°, respectively (Fig. 3.22).

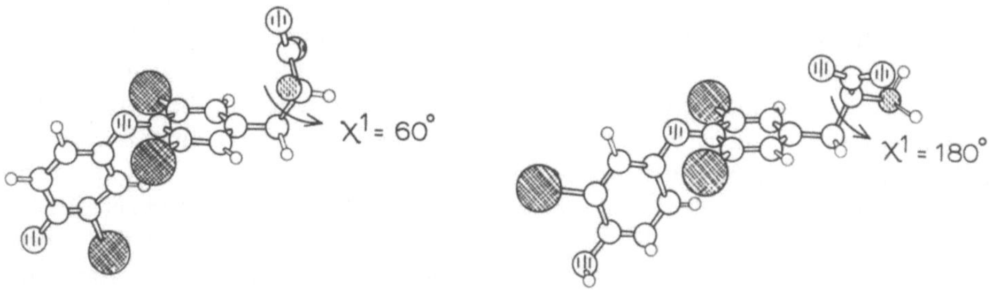

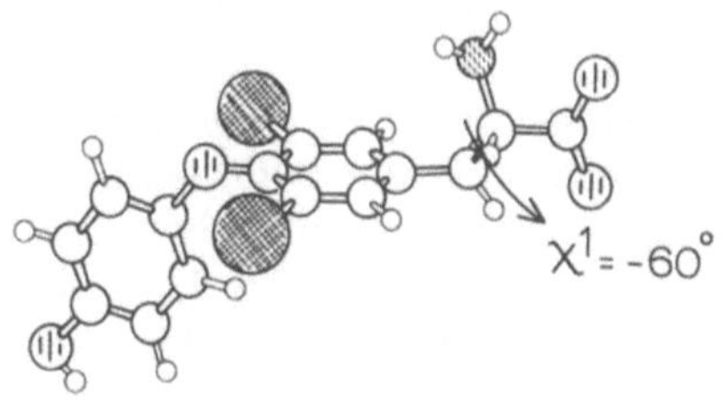

Fig. 3.21. An illustration of the amino acid conformation χ^1 (C1-C7-C8-N8) at 60°, 180°, and −60°

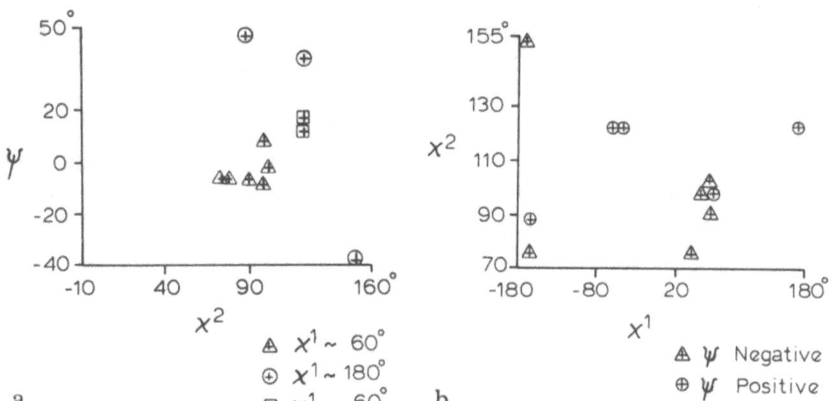

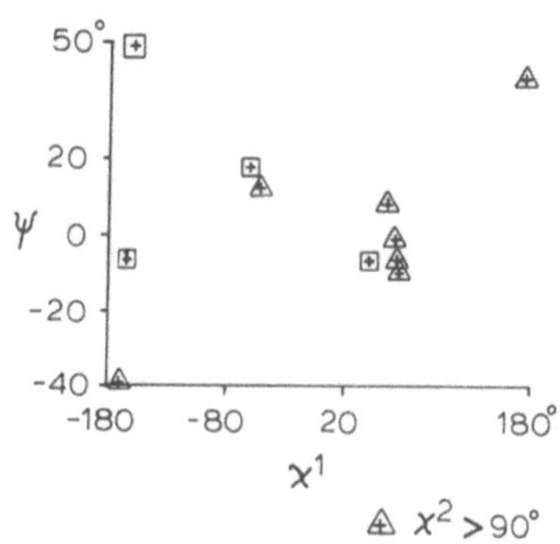

c

Fig. 3.22 a–c. Possible correlations among the amino acid parameters χ^2, χ^1 and ψ for those thyronine derivatives in Table 3.1. **a** A plot of χ^2 versus ψ showing that those structures with $\chi^1 = 60°$, χ^2 and ψ fall near their ideal values of 90° and 0°, respectively; **b** plot of χ^2 versus χ^1, no correlations; **c** A plot of χ^1 versus ψ, no correlations

A value of $\chi^1 = 180°$ (Fig. 3.21) has the amine function fully extended with respect to the inner ring. This is a more favorable energy minimum than $\chi^1 = 60°$. In this orientation the amine could hydrogen bond to receptor functional groups with a minimum of steric interference of the diphenyl–ether portion of the molecule.

A similar situation is presented when $\chi^1 = -60°$ (Fig. 3.21). In this case the carboxylic function is fully extended with respect to the inner ring and again the same potential to hydrogen bond is present as in the $\chi^1 = 180°$ case. The net effect of these three energy minima is illustrated in Fig. 3.23 which shows the superimposition of all three on the C7–C8 bond. As will be seen, these considerations are of major importance in describing the thyroxine–prealbumin interactions (Andrea 1977).

Amino acid side chain conformations also have been studied using empirical molecular orbital (MO) methods (Dietrich 1976). In these calculations χ^1 and χ^2 were varied systematically with ψ set at $-15°$. These studies led to the local energy minima shown in Table 3.5, which are compared with the observed average values from crystallographic observations. As can be noted, χ^1 values are in good agreement, but those for χ^2 differ greatly.

The greatest differences are observed for those structures with $\chi^1 = -60°$. The net effect of this change in χ^2 (Fig. 3.24) is a shift in the side chain orientation with respect to that of the inner ring. This movement from $\chi^2 = 121°$ to $\chi^2 = 75°$ produces an N8 . . . H2 constant distance of 2.66 Å (Table 3.6), the Van der Waals radii for these two atoms. Normally this contact distance is near 4.00 Å. Thus, there are no obvious structural reasons for the disparity of these results. In addition to these local energy minima, two steep minima were observed at $\chi^2 = 60°$, $\chi^1 = 210°$; $\chi^2 = 240°$, $\chi^1 = 210°$. Dietrich attributed these minima to an attractive interaction between the functional groups and H2 and H6 of the ring, and considered them an artifact of the approximations in the CNDO/2 MO method.

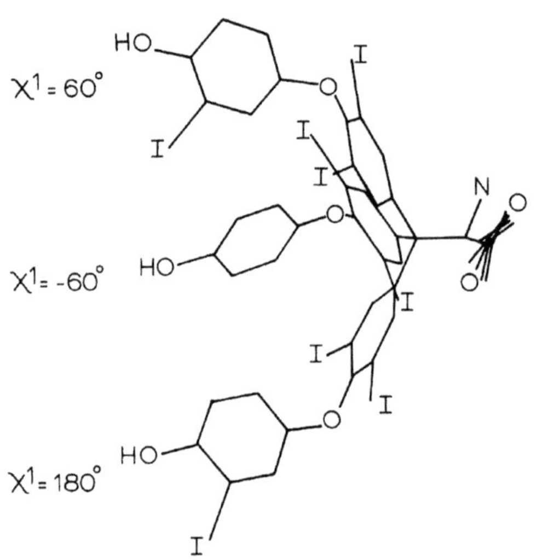

Fig. 3.23. A superimposition of thyroid structures showing $\chi^1 = 60°$, 180°, and $-60°$

Table 3.5. Amino acid side chain conformation

Conformation	χ^1	χ^2	ψ
Average crystal structure[a]	59°	94°	− 3°
Predicted MO energy values[b]	60	105	−15
Crystal	190	109	10
MO	180	90	−15
Crystal	− 56	121	15
MO	− 60	75	−15

[a] Average of values for thyronines listed in Table 3.1.
[b] Predicted energy minimum molecular orbital conformation.
(Dietrich 1976, p 189)

However, the results of crystallographic studies indicate that this extra stabilization energy need not be attributed to approximation errors in the MO calculations. An analysis of the amino acid structures (Table 3.6) shows that there are 3.0 Å distances between the functional groups (N8, O9, O10) and the inner ring hydrogens. In the case of χ^1 near 60°, both the N8 and O10 groups remain 3.0 Å distant from both H2 and H6. When χ^1 is near 180°, only O9 maintains this distance while for χ^1 near −60°, N8 has a close approach, but this time nearer to 3.8 Å. All of these contact distances are greater than the sum of the Van der Waals radii for these atoms and, thus, do not contribute extra stabilization energy.

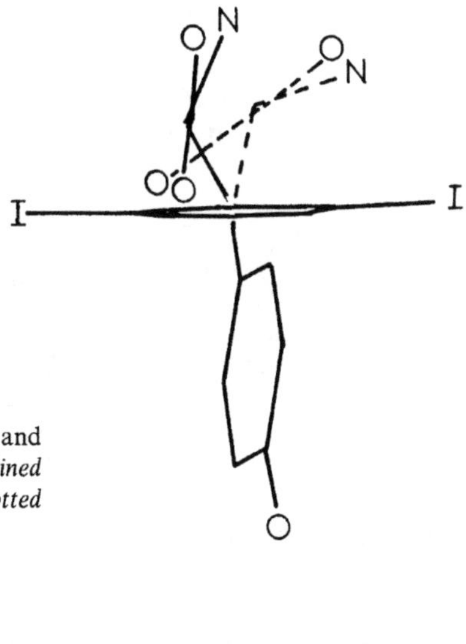

Fig. 3.24. Comparison between observed crystal structure and MO energy calculated model for χ^2 conformation. *Solid lined* molecule is X-ray structure $\chi^2 = 120°$, $\chi^1 = -59°$ and the *dotted lined* molecule is $\chi^2 = 75°$, $\chi^1 = 60°$ (Table 3.5)

Table 3.6. Amino acid intramolecular contacts

Structure	χ^1	χ^2	H2–N8	H2–O9	H2–O10	H6–N8	H6–O9	H6–O10
TO07	56°	98°	3.00 Å	5.33 Å	5.01 Å	4.09 Å	4.58 Å	3.00 Å
TO05	−164	76	4.87	3.20	4.38	4.38	4.36	5.60
TO01	− 59	121	3.76	4.55	5.29	3.83	5.22	5.59
TO01[a]	− 59	75	4.65	4.65	5.92	2.66	5.14	4.92

[a] Conformation set to molecular orbit (MO) calculated minimum, Table 3.5.

If it is assumed that the amino acid end of the molecule is of primary importance to a binding site (or, as in thyroglobulin, where the hormone is part of the polypeptide backbone) then the consequence of changes in χ^1 would be dramatic. However, these same changes would appear more subtle if the diphenyl ether end of the molecule were assumed fixed by a receptor. Therefore, changes in relative binding affinities for the thyroid hormones and their analogues to receptors ultimately depend on the specific steric requirements of the receptor site and the ability of the hormone to adopt the required conformation. Also, differences in relative binding affinities among the binding proteins reflect the changes in structural characteristics needed for binding. In addition to conformation, the net charge of the side chain could play an important role in binding ability.

IV. Intermolecular Interactions

In addition to understanding of molecular conformation derived from an analysis of the five rotational parameters defining the thyronine nucleus, it is important to understand how these molecules interact with their environment. This can be achieved, to some measure, by an analysis of the crystallographic packing arrangement of the molecules in the lattice. As shown (Fig. 3.25), there are several potential hydrogen bond donor and acceptor sites on the thyronine nucleus. Under normal physiologic conditions, the amino acid is a zwitterion with the amine having a net positive charge and the carboxylic oxygens a net negative charge. Also, the 4′-OH can act as a hydrogen bond donor or acceptor. In addition, at physiologic pH, T_4 is about 80% ionized, whereas in T_3 this group is almost 90% in the unionized form (Korcek and Tabachnick 1976).

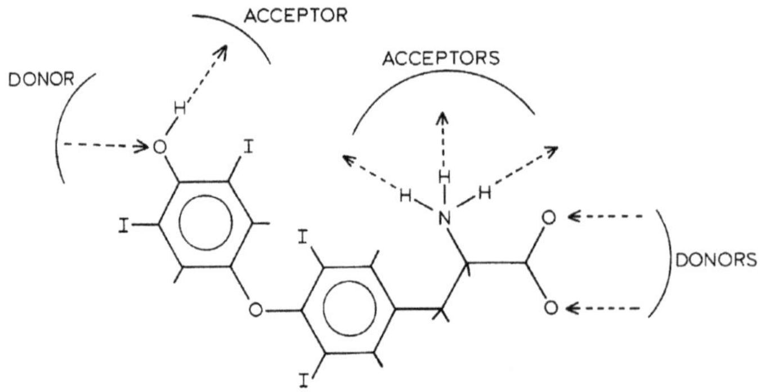

Fig. 3.25. Hydrogen bond interactions in thyroxine

A hydrogen bond is usually viewed in terms of the three directly participating atoms: D, the donor atom; A, the acceptor; and the hydrogen atom D–H . . . A, where H . . . . A is the hydrogen bond itself. Whether or not a particular arrangement of atoms represents a hydrogen bond is dependent upon the complete geometric description of the arrangement, i. e., the distances, D–H, H . . . . A and the angle D–H . . . . . A. Specifically, the H . . . . A separation should be shorter than the sum of Van der Waals radii[2] of the hydrogen and acceptor atom (Baur 1972).

A study of the hydrogen bonding patterns in these thyroactive structures indicates a high degree of directional specificity in the location of hydrogen bond donors and acceptors. In general, the thyroid hormone structures tend to line up head (4′-OH) to tail (amino acid) where the phenyl hydroxyl is hydrogen bonded to the amino acid of the next molecule in line (Fig. 3.26 a). When organic solvent molecules cocrystallize with the thyroactive compound, they tend to share the hydrogen bonding with the amine rather than disrupt the overall pattern. However, in a few cases, the molecules form layers with a head to head or tail to tail alignment in each layer. When there is water and HCl in the lattice, these tend to form channels through the lattice separating the layers of tail to tail hydrogen bonding between the thyroactive molecules (Fig. 3.26 b).

In those structures in which the 4′-OH acts as a hydrogen bond donor (Table 3.7, Fig. 3.27), the acceptor atom is a carboxylic oxygen from an adjacent molecule in the lattice. The acceptor atoms approach the 4′-OH from directions nearly coplanar with the phenoxy ring plane (C3′-C4′-O4′1 . . . X) and at an angle (C4′-O41′ . . . X) of 120°. In addition, for T_3 structures, the direction of approach is trans to the 3′-iodine, whether distal or proximal. When the 4′-OH acts as a hydrogen bond acceptor, the donor atoms (Table 3.7) tend to approach the phenoxy ring from directions either above or below the plane and opposite the acceptor atom (Fig. 3.28).

As presented in Table 3.7, the average value for the hydrogen bond angle C4-O4′1 . . . X is 116° when the 4′-OH acts as a donor and 129° when it is an acceptor. Also, when the 4′-OH is simultaneously involved as a donor and acceptor, the donor atom to 4′-OH tends to have an angle near 150°. When the hydrogen bonding atoms are water, one adopts the orientation observed for the carboxylic oxygens, suggesting that it is a hydrogen bond acceptor from the 4′-OH.

In the case of tetraiodothyroactive structures in which the 4′-oxygen is a phenoxide ion (Cody 1978 a) and thus only a hydrogen bond acceptor, the donor atoms approach the 4′-phenoxy ring symmetrically from directions both above and below the plane (Fig. 3.28 c). However, where the tetraiodo structures are hydroxyls (T_4A) (Cody et al. 1977 a, b), the outer ring iodines cause the approach of the donor/acceptor atoms to deviate from this pattern.

A study of the 4′-O . . . X hydrogen bonds in these structures shows that the average O . . . O distance is 2.74 Å and the O . . . N distance is 2.76 Å, which is in general agreement with other studies (Mitra and Ramakrishnan, 1977). When the

2 The Van der Waals radius of an atom makes an allowance both for the volume occupied by the atom and for the attractive force between the atoms. Van der Waals forces are attractive in nature and thus the radius measures the closest approach of two atoms before their orbital electrons begin to repel one another. Therefore, Van der Waals radii for all elements may be estimated if the distances of closest approach of their atoms to one another, when no chemical bond exists between them, are known from structural studies.

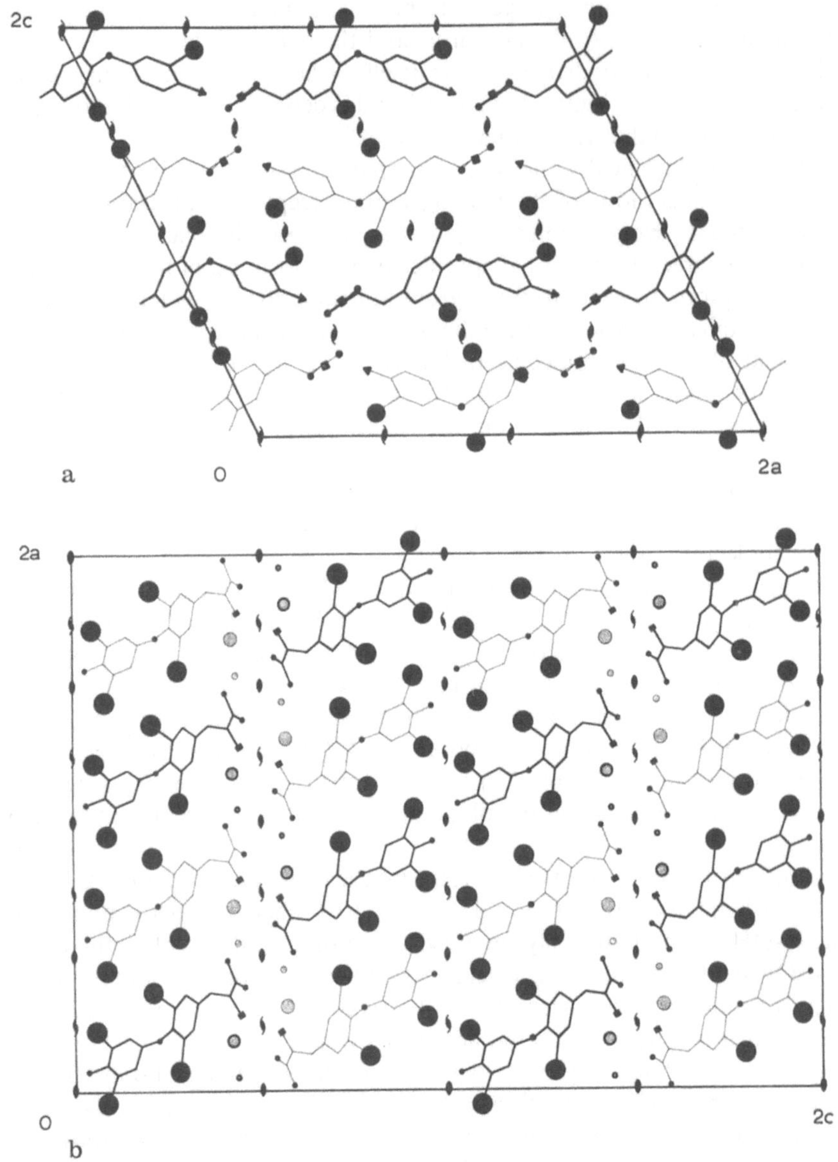

Fig. 3.26. a Crystal packing arrangement of T_3 (TO05, Table 3.1) in its crystal lattice projected down the lattice b-axis. The dark molecules are viewed above the light ones; the large circles are iodine, small circles are oxygen, the triangles are hydroxyls, and the squares are nitrogen. **b** Crystal packing arrangement of T_4 (TO09, Table 3.1) in its crystal lattice projected down the lattice b-axis. The dark molecules are viewed above the light ones, the large filled circles are iodine, the large stippled ones are chlorine, the small filled circles are oxygen, the small open circles are water, and the squares are nitrogen

donor and acceptor O . . . O values are considered separately, these become 2.66 Å and 2.81 Å for 4′-OH as a donor and acceptor, respectively.

The results of theoretical energy calculations of inter- and intramolecular hydrogen bond strengths of ortho-substituted phenol and phenoxides (Andrea et al.

(Text continued p. 41)

Table 3.7. Hydrogen bond directionality in thyroactive structures

Structure	4′-OH as donor				4′-OH as acceptor			
	X	C3′–C4′–O4′1…X	C4′–O4′1…X	O…X	X	C3′–C4′–O4′1…X	C4′–O4′1…X	O…X
Diiodothyronine (TO01)[a]	09	−175°	108°	2.62 Å	N4	38°	124°	2.97 Å
					N8	−77	116	2.04
Dibromothyroacetic acid (TO11)	08	162	119	2.59				
Diiodothyropropionic acid (TO12)	010	−177	118	2.82				
Triiodothyronine methyl ester (TO03)					N8	168	126	2.69
Triiodothyroacetic acid (TO04)	09	−176	119	2.59	07	33	145	3.02
Triiodothyronine (TO05)	09	151	124	2.63	N8	−10	151	2.82
Triiodothyronine, HCl, H_2O (TO07)					02	108	127	2.68
					03	176	119	2.69
Triiodothyropropionic acid ethyl ester (TO08)	09	160	115	2.75				
2′,3′-Dimethyl-diiodothyronine H_2O (TO15)					01	−94	113	3.17
					02	49	137	2.51
3′-Isopropyl-diiodothyronine H_2O (TO10)					01	−83	127	2.51
					01	−6	127	2.73
Thyroxine, HCl, H_2O (TO09)					04′1	−25	145	2.91
Tetraiodothyroacetic acid (TO13)	09	118	108	2.59	07A	178	150	3.08
Tetraiodothyroformic acid (TO14)					N4A	89	132	2.71
					N4B	−78	118	2.70
Thyroxine (TO16) A					N8A	73	113	2.65
					N44	−102	134	2.60
B					N8B	73	113	2.65
					N43	109	130	2.70

[a] These numbers refer to the listing in Table 3.1.

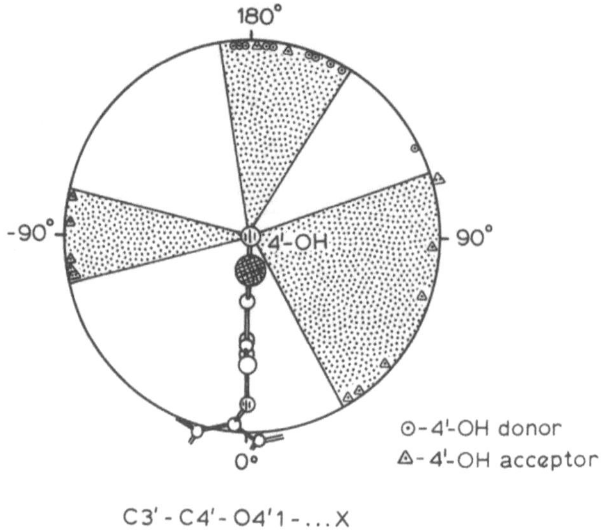

Fig. 3.27. Distribution of hydrogen bond directionality with 4'-OH as acceptor and donor. Plot is hydrogen bond torsion angle C3'-C4'-O4'1 . . . χ

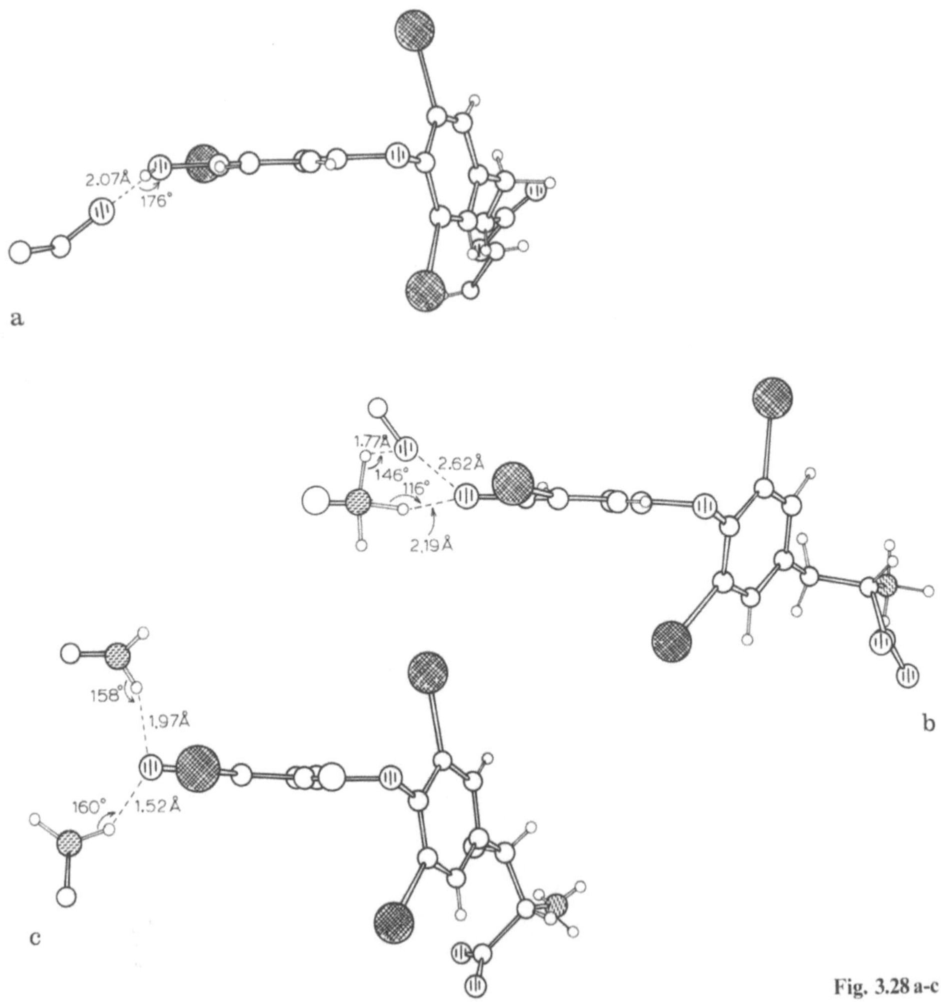

Fig. 3.28 a-c

1979), as models to investigate likely orientations of thyroid hormones at their protein binding sites, are in general agreement with the hydrogen bonding patterns observed in these crystallographic determinations. These energy calculations predict an average O . . . O distance of 2.63 Å and a C-O . . . O angle of 125°, irrespective of whether the 4′-OH is acting as a proton donor or acceptor. Unfortunately, this study (Andrea et al. 1979) did not compute the hydrogen bond geometry when the 4′-OH is simultaneously acting as a hydrogen bond donor and acceptor, and, consequently, the detail observed from the crystallographic data is not apparent.

The observation that in the 3′-substituted structures the hydrogen bonding atom approaches the 4′-OH trans to the 3′-substituent is verification of quantitative structure activity relationship (QSAR) data which also suggest that in vitro binding of T_3 probably involves hydrogen bond donation of the 4′-OH to the 5′-side of the nuclear receptor (Dietrich 1976).

The amine acts as a hydrogen bond donor to oxygen except in those structures which contain HCl, where it then hydrogen bonds to the Cl^-. When there are solvent molecules in the lattice, they will generally hydrogen bond to the amine nitrogen.

The hydrogen bond patterns observed in these crystal structures can be used as models for hormone–receptor interactions. In this case, the local environment at the various hydrogen bond sites (i. e., 4′-OH, NH_3^+, COO^-) can be interpreted in terms of potential hydrogen bond interactions with appropriate side chain groups in the backbone of the serum or nuclear proteins.

For example, the NH_3^+ group of lysine or arginine could act as a hydrogen bond donor to the 4′-phenoxide of T_4 or the 4′-OH of T_3, as represented in Figs. 3.28 b and 3.28 c. Also, the acid group of aspartic or glutamic acid could function as a hydrogen bond acceptor from the 4′-OH or NH_3^+ of the hormone molecule. Such side chains as serine, threonine, tyrosine, or hydroxyproline, each with an available hydroxyl, could interact either as hydrogen bond donors or acceptors to an appropriate hormone-functional group. The facilitation of any of these situations depends on the pH at the local binding environment.

D. Role of Iodine in Conformation and Activity

Since the thyroid hormones are the only naturally occurring iodinated compounds known to have vital biochemical activity, it is presumed that iodine plays an essential role in hormone activity. Some investigators have proposed that enhanced thyroid activity may be related to the ability of iodine to (1) achieve and maintain a specific hormone conformation or (2) direct electronic interactions such as charge-transfer or electron-donor effects in molecular associations. Recent studies on the

◀ **Fig. 3.28. a** T_3P (TO08, Table 3.1) 4′-OH hydrogen bond geometry showing the direction of approach of a hydrogen bond acceptor. (Only a fragment of the acceptor molecule is shown.) **b** T_3 (TO05, Table 3.1) 4′-OH hydrogen bond geometry showing the directions of approach of both hydrogen bond donor and acceptor. **c** Thyroxine (TO16A1, Table 3.1) 4′–O hydrogen bond geometry showing directions of approach of the hydrogen bond donors

activity and binding properties of halogen-free thyronine analogues (Jorgensen et al. 1974; Snyder et al. 1976) imply a distinction between these proposed functional roles of iodine and throw light on their significance for hormonal activity.

I. Conformational Constraints

One of the primary roles assigned to the inner ring iodines is that of maintaining a skewed or twist-skewed diphenyl-ether conformation. This conformational constraint is illustrated in Fig. 3.29, which compares the diphenyl-ether conformation of thyronine ethyl ester (TO06) (Table 3.1) with that of 3,5-diiodothyronine (TO01) (Table 3.1). Here the bulky ortho iodines appear to provide the steric constraints necessary to stabilize this arrangement as an energy minimum conformation. The analysis of the methyl analogue of T_3 (TO18) (Table 3.1) permits a comparison of the relative influence of iodine and methyl substituents upon thyronine conformation. The observation of a twist-skewed, distal 3′-methyl conformation for this trimethyl thyronine analogue (Cody 1978 b) (Fig. 3.30) indicates that methyl substituents have sufficient bulk to maintain this perpendicular arrangement of the phenyl rings. As illustrated in Fig. 3.30 b, the diphenyl ether conformation of the trimethyl analogue is almost indistinguishable from that of the hormone T_3 as its methyl ester. These data reemphasize the steric specificity of the thyromimetic compound for activity.

In general, the diphenyl ethers that have no 3,5-substituents have conformations similar to that of thyronine, while all other 3,5-substituents (Me, Cl, isoproyl, *t*-butyl) maintain a perpendicular ring conformation (Van der Heijden et al. 1975).

II. Electronic Effects

In addition to providing a bulkiness that would force a specific conformation, the inner ring iodines may interact with the transport proteins via a charge-transfer mechanism (Mauchamp and Shinitzky 1969; Cilento 1975). It has been shown that charge-transfer forces may contribute to the association of two or more molecules. Similar to other types of associations, charge-transfer complexing may influence equilibrium and reactivity and is in turn influenced by pH and solvent effects. Charge-transfer associations can be either inter- or intramolecular in nature.

It had been suggested (Cilento and Berenholc 1965) that thyroxine may act in intermolecular energy-transfer reactions by being able to capture the energy of

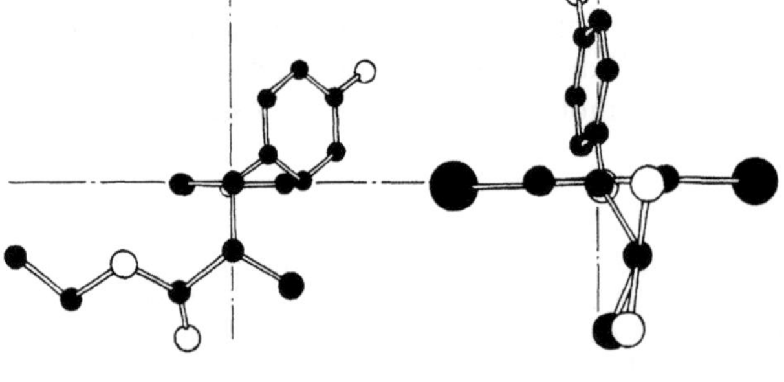

Fig. 3.29. Comparison of the conformation of thyronine ethyl ester (TO06, Table 3.1) with diiodothyronine (TO01). This view is projected down the vector from C1 to C4 of the inner phenyl ring. (Cody 1978 a)

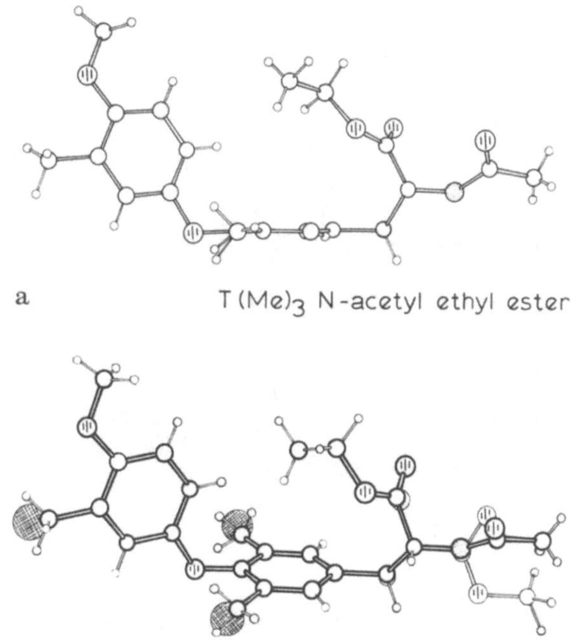

Fig. 3.30. **a** Conformation of the trimethylthyronine derivative (TO18, Table 3.1); **b** superimposition of TO18 with that of T_3Me (TO03, Table 3.1)

excited state products of biologic reactions to form molecular complexes with other biologically important components. However, these proposals of iodine activity by perturbation effects were questioned when recent data showed nonhalogen thyroxine analogues to possess activity (Jorgensen et al. 1974; Jorgensen 1976; Ramsden 1975). Also by this theory, mono- and diiodotyrosine should possess activity, but they do not.

The idea of conformational restrictions in combination with iodine-perturbation effects was also proposed as a necessary prerequisite for thyromimetic activity. Lehmann (1972, 1974) proposed that an intramolecular charge-transfer complex exists in thyroid hormone structures which is responsible for maintaining conformational rigidity. This proposed energy minimum conformation (Fig. 3.31) places one of the inner ring iodines above the outer phenyl ring, forming an intramolecular π-complex.

According to Lehmann (1972), this proposed twist conformation ($\varphi=217°$; $\varphi'=37°$) places one inner ring iodine directly over the C1′ atom (I . . . C1′ = 3.5 Å), thereby placing the iodine outer orbitals in the densest part of the outer ring π-electron cloud. However, as can be seen from Fig. 3.13, the 3.5 Å distance is a constant feature of the perpendicular conformation and yet does not reflect any π overlap. Moreover, a much better π-intramolecular charge-transfer complex would exist in the case of an "anti-skewed" structure (Table 3.2) which, by reversing the values of φ and φ', places the inner iodine atom directly over the outer ring (2.1 Å). There is, however, no solid state evidence for this type of intramolecular charge-transfer complex or of a stable twist conformation (Table 3.1). On the other hand,

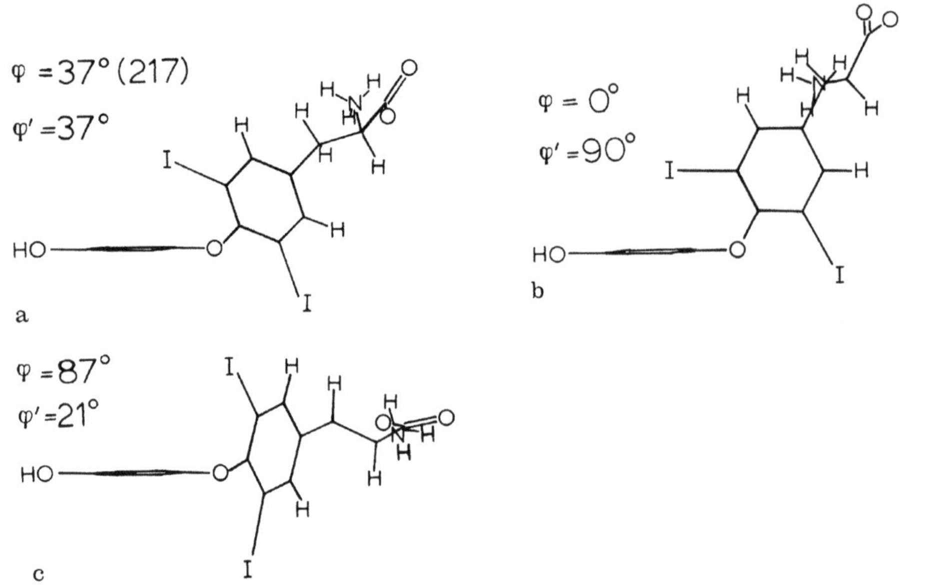

Fig. 3.31. a Proposed intramolecular charge-transfer model for T_3 showing a diphenyl ether conformation of $\varphi = 37°$, $\varphi' = 37°$. **b** Proposed antiskewed diphenyl ether model for T_3 ($\varphi = 0°$, $\varphi' = 90°$) with intramolecular charge-transfer between the inner ring iodine and the outer ring. **c** Observed twist-skewed conformation of TO01 (Table 3.1)

there are numerous examples of unusually close iodine intermolecular Van der Waals contacts to other iodine and oxygen atoms in the crystal lattice.

III. Iodine Interactions

There are two commonly accepted values for the Van der Waals radii of iodine and oxygen. The values reported by Bondi (1964) for iodine (1.98 Å) and oxygen (1.50 Å) are more compatible with experimental density data than the frequently quoted Van der Waals radii based on Pauling's (1960) approximations (I = 2.15 Å, O = 1.40 Å). From these considerations then, the closest approach of two nonbonded iodine atoms would be 4.30 Å or 3.96 Å depending on whose values were used. Similarly, the iodine–oxygen approaches would be 3.55 Å or 3.50 Å.

One measure of the polarizability and charge-transfer ability of the iodine atom is the observation of a large number of short intermolecular contact distances of the type I . . . I and I . . . O in the crystal lattice. An analysis of these intermolecular contacts reveals that the average I . . . I distance is 4.00 Å based on 32 observations in 13 different crystal structures. The corresponding I . . . O average is 3.19 Å based on ten observations in eight crystal structures. The I . . . I values range from 3.69 Å to 4.29 Å whereas the I . . . O values range from 2.99 Å to 3.45 Å.

Examination of the data shows that it is predominantly the inner ring iodine atoms which participate in these interactions. This property may explain the observation that the two inner ring iodine atoms are of greater importance for binding than the outer ring iodines (Jorgensen 1976; Hao and Tabachnick 1971).

Activity measurements of various 3,5-substituted analogues of T_4 (Jorgensen, 1976) have shown that symmetric, lipophilic groups, not exceeding iodine in size, are required to maintain significant hormonal response. These studies also indicate that the size constraints of the 3,5-substituents may be more important for activity than their lipophilic character (Pittman and Pittman 1974; Murray 1974). However, there is a good correlation between biologic activity and the lipophilic and electron-donor characteristics of substituents on the outer ring. Thus, 3′-isoproyl-3, 5-diiodothyronine is highly active while 3′-iodo-3,5-diisopropylthyronine possesses almost no activity.

These differences in activity with comparable substitution in either the inner or outer phenyl ring have led some investigators to suggest that the 3,5-diiodotyrosyl moiety is associated with the transport and the receptor binding of T_4 and that the outer phenyl ring imparts the functional activity of T_4 (Pittman and Pittman 1974).

The importane of conformational fit with the receptor as a determining factor for biologic activity is suggested by the observation that activity follows the order $I > Br > CH_3 > Cl > F > H$ for 3,5-substitution (Murray 1974). Also, only those groups that can maintain a skewed-ring system possess biologic activity. Another important factor may be "dispersion-force" binding of the 3,5 groups to points on the receptor surface, which again would follow the activity order cited above.

Therefore, in addition to maintaining a specific hormone conformation, the inner ring iodines, by nature of their polarizability, may also have a significant role in receptor binding to a hydrophobic surface with close tolerances for fit. Thus, one could envision the inner ring presenting a "polarized" surface to the receptor, which then adheres to the receptor, somewhat like Velcro. Those functional groups that can both maintain the proper conformation and present the proper adhesive surface have high binding affinities to the transport proteins.

IV. Acidity 4′-OH

Another effect of iodine substitution in thyroid hormones is the observation that the acidity of the 4′-OH increases with ortho-iodine substitution, as is indicated by the pKa values for T_2, T_3, and T_4 of 10.0, 8.47, 6.73, respectively. This acidity difference between T_3 and T_4 has been proposed as one factor governing activity since at physiologic pH (7.3–7.4), the phenolic hydroxyl of T_4 is about 80% ionized whereas in T_3 this group is almost 90% in the un-ionized form (Korcek and Tabachnick 1976). Not only is the binding of T_4 analogues to the serum proteins strongly influenced by the degree of 4′-OH ionization, but it is apparently the 4′-phenoxide ion which enhances binding to serum proteins (Snyder et al. 1976). These binding data also suggest that an un-ionized 4′-OH is more likely for nuclear binding receptor interactions.

To identify any differences in geometry and conformation between T_3 and T_4 and their influence on binding and activity, a comparison of the crystal structures of T_3 and T_4 was undertaken. This comparative study reveals that there are significant differences between tetra- and triiodothyroactive structures which are compatible with the increased acidity of the thyroxine 4′-OH group. As illustrated in Fig. 3.32, there are several significant differences in the outer phenyl ring-geometry. The values shown in this figure are the average values obtained from six T_3 structures

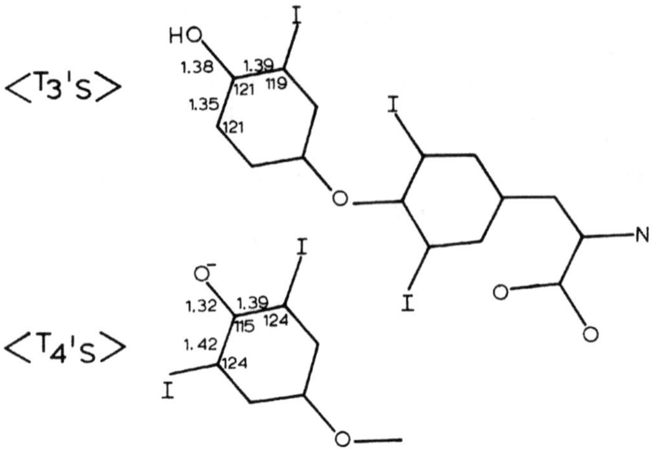

Fig. 3.32. Electronic and geometric differences in the outer phenyl ring of a series of T_4 and T_3 structures. These values represent an average of six T_3 and three T_4 structures, respectively. The average standard deviations on the bond and angles in these structures are less than 0.02 Å and 1.0°, respectively. Standard aromatic values are C–OH, 1.38 Å; C=O, 1.30 Å; C–C, 1.39 Å, C–C–C, 120°. (Cody 1978 a)

(TO03,4,5,7,8,17) (Table 3.2) and three T_4 structures[3] (TO14, 16A, B), only those average values that differed significantly are reported here.

These results show that for the thyroxine 4′-phenoxide ion there is a contraction of the C3′-C4′-C5′ angle, a slight increase in the bonds adjacent to the C4′ atom and an expansion of the carbon angles at both C3′ and C5′ positions when compared with the 4′-hydroxyl T_3 structures. No changes are observed in the C–I bond lengths. The expected values for these parameters are as follows: C–OH 1.38 Å, C=O 1.30 Å, C–C 1.39 Å, C–C–C 120°. These changes in geometry are significantly greater than the estimated standard deviations reported from their individual structure determinations which range from 0.003 to 0.02 Å and from 0.4 to 1.0°. In each of these T_4 structures, the thyroactive compounds form a complex with the base *N*-diethanolamine, each forming a strong O . . . N hydrogen bond in which the nitrogen is the hydrogen-bond donor.

These results showing 4′-phenoxide ion formation and the associated differences between T_4 and T_3 structures verify theoretical energy models and protein-binding studies (Dietrich et al. 1977) which show that the 3′ and 5′ substituents influence the degree of plasma protein binding. These data also suggest that it is apparently the 4′-phenoxide which binds to the plasma protein TBG whereas the nuclear receptor binds as un-ionized 4′-OH in T_3.

E. Protein Binding and Biologic Activity

The thyroid hormones bind three classes of receptor: (1) plasma proteins which transport the hormones through the general circulation; (2) membrane-bound proteins which interact with the hormones at the cell surface; and (3) nuclear

3 The results of TO02 and TO09 were not used in this computation.

proteins through which hormonal activity is expressed. There are three thyroid specific proteins in the plasma: TBG, which carries about 75% of the hormones; TBPA, which carries about 15% of the hormones, and human serum albumin (HSA), which transports the rest (see Chap. 2). These serum proteins may function as a buffer responsible for keeping a large store of thyroid hormones in the extrathyroidal space in a nondiffusible form, and/or they may act as donors of hormones from the microcirculation to the cells (Robbins 1975).

Receptor proteins that may mediate thyroid hormone action have been found in varying amounts in mitochondrial membranes, cytosol. and nonhistone chromatin fractions of several hormone-responsive tissues (Oppenheimer et al. 1974; Samuels and Tsai 1974; Spindler et al. 1975; DeGroot and Torresani 1975; Sterling et al. 1977). Physicochemical studies show that a major nuclear T_3-binding component has a Stokes radius of 33 Å, a sedimentation coefficient of 3.5S, and a mol. wt. from 48 000 to 65 000 (Torresani et al. 1978; Surks et al. 1973 b; Surks and Oppenheimer 1976).

Interactions of thyroid hormones with nuclear receptors appear not to require an intermediate cytoplasmic receptor. Instead, the hormones bind directly to receptors that are permanent residents in the nuclear chromatin (Clark et al. 1976). Cytosol-T_3 proteins may regulate the free T_3 concentration in the cell and thus influence the distribution of the hormone in other cellular compartments.

Recent evidence (Samuels et al. 1977) also indicates that there are two components of nuclear-bound receptors having different half-lives in the presence of T_3: a hormone-depletable component which consists of 40%–50% of the receptor population and a relatively nondepletable receptor component. This study implies that the nuclear receptor may associate with different components that may have different regulatory functions. Furthermore, the good correlation between thyromimetic potency and binding affinities supports the concept that these sites are the points of initiation of hormonal response (Oppenheimer et al. 1975 a).

In addition to these findings, mitochondrial-binding proteins specific to the thyroid hormones have been identified (Sterling and Milch 1975; Sterling et al. 1977, 1978; Singh et al. 1976; Holm et al. 1977). Proteins from the inner mitochondrial membrane were found to possess high affinities for the thyroid hormones with stereospecific discrimination between L- and D-T_4 (Table 3.8). Analogue-binding affinities were also related to their known physiologic potencies (Singh et al. 1976; Sterling et al. 1977).

Further evidence for a role of the cell surface in the thyroid hormone uptake was observed in studies with rat liver plasma membranes, in which high affinity binding sites for thyroid hormones were detected (Holm et al. 1977). These studies show that the thyroid hormones must interact with specific plasma membrane structures in order to enter target cells and then bind to intracellular components. Thus, the role of nuclear sites in restraining the response to thyroid hormone administration emphasizes that the mechanism of hormone delivery to the nuclei is critical in determining hormonal response (Oppenheimer et al. 1976).

Protein binding is therefore central to the transport, tissue distribution, and metabolism rates of the various thyroid analogues (Pittman and Pittman 1974) and, because of this, the ease of metabolism and the availability of the hormones to various body compartments are governed by the strength of protein binding. Current theory proposes that (1) the hormone binds a specific site on the

Table 3.8. Relative binding affinities and biologic potencies of selected thyroid hormones and their analogues to serum and nuclear proteins

Compound	TBG (Snyder et al. 1976)	Nuclear (Jorgensen 1978)	Membrane (Singh et al. 1976)	Potency (Jorgensen 1978)
L-Thyroxine	100.0%	12.5%	96.6%	12.5%
D-Thyroxine	54.0	–	63.0	–
N-Acetyl thyroxine	25.0	–	–	–
Tetraiodothyropropionic acid	3.6	–	23.0	1.9
Tetraiodothyroacetic acid	1.7	–	30.3	6.25
S-Bridge thyroxine	63.0	–	–	–
CH_2-Bridge thyroxine	35.0	2.6	–	–
3′,5′-Diiodo-3,5-dibromo-DL-thyronine	161.0	–	54.2	–
Tetrabromo-DL-thyronine	40.0	–	–	–
Tetramethylthyronine	0.0	0.1	–	0.3
2′,3′-Dimethyl-3,5-diiodothyronine	0.71	1.1	–	6.3
2′,5′-Dimethyl-3,5-diiodothyronine	0.13	0.1	–	0.1
L-3,5,3′-Triiodothyronine	9.0	100.0	100.0	100.0
3′,5′,3-Triiodothyronine	38.0	0.1	67.5	<0.1
Triiodothyroacetic acid	0.3	–	60.6	4.4
3,5,3′-Tribromothyronine	6.2	–	46.5	–
3′,5′,3-Tribromothyronine	6.5	–	–	–
S-Bridge triiodothyronine	13.0	100.0	–	29.0
Trimethylthyronine	–	0.1	–	0.4
3,3′-Diiodothyronine	1.3	0.5	–	0.0
3′,5′-Diiodothyronine	0.1	–	–	–
3,5-Diiodothyronine	0.07	0.3	60.6	1.2
3-Monoiodothyronine	0.05	–	35.3	–
3′-Monoiodothyronine	0.023	–	–	–
Thyronine	0.0	–	25.4	–

macromolecular receptor, and (2) an interaction takes place between some chemically reactive feature of the hormone and a complementary component on the receptor. Steric correspondence between the receptor site and the hormone then permits electronic interaction. Thus, the structural specificity of the hormone can be both steric and electronic in nature.

The activity and binding affinities of analogues that differ from the natural hormones in only a single structural feature serve to identify the contribution of that feature to the production of hormonal effects. These analyses can also serve as probes to describe the hormone-receptor interactions at an active site (Jorgensen 1978).

The multiplicity of physiologic effects caused by the thyroid hormones has given rise to a variety of assay systems that may be used to measure the relative potencies of the hormones and their analogues. Tests with rat antigoiter, rat oxygen consumption, and tadpole metamorphis tests have been most widely used to determine the relative activities of thyroid hormone analogues in vivo (Jorgensen

1976, 1978). Recent studies using intact cells and hormone-binding studies with subcellular components have also led to relative thyroid hormone analogue potencies in in vitro systems.

Numerous studies measuring the relative binding affinities of the hormones and their analogues for these serum and nuclear proteins have been carried out (Hao and Tabachnick 1971; Tabachnick and Korcek 1978; Koerner et al. 1975; Goldfine et al. 1976; Snyder et al. 1976; Surks and Oppenheimer 1976; Jorgensen 1978; Bolger 1978) and the results indicate the importance of specific structural features in binding. These studies show that the receptor-hormone interaction sites on these proteins differ as the structural features important for maximal binding differ.

Table 3.8 lists a few of the activity and binding affinity data available for the thyroid hormones and their analogues. Because there is a large data base of structurally similar compounds available, a number of attempts to define the quantitative structure-activity relationships (QSAR) governing properties such as steric hindrance, lipophilicity, or electronic effects have been carried out (Kubinyi 1976; Dietrich et al. 1977). On the basis of these studies the concept of the hormone molecule acting as a structurally specific matrix was developed as opposed to a particular functional portion of the molecule being involved in hormone action. In general, the results of these QSAR studies indicated that these parameters are reasonable estimates of the physical properties they are designed to predict. Thus, in addition to describing observed characteristics, these parameters can be used to design new thyroactive compounds.

I. Nuclear Binding Proteins

Structural requirements for potency (Table 3.8) correlate closely with those for in vitro binding to nuclear proteins (Jorgensen 1978). These correlations, in conjunction with other thyroid hormone studies, provide the following general description of structural features for both in vivo hormonal activity and for association to the T_3-receptor sites of cell nuclei.

1) A central lipophilic core of two mutually perpendicular aromatic rings with a bridging (O,S,C) atom at a 120° angle.
2) Nonpolar groups (halogen, methyl) in the 3,5-positions, providing size-limited hydrophobic binding interactions with the receptor.
3) Specific polar groups in the 1-position and a 4′-phenolic hydroxyl group are required at opposite ends of the central diphenyl ether core.
4) Activity of this primary structure is enhanced by a single lipophilic substituent (halogen, alkyl) in the distal 3′-position.
5) A second proximal 5′-lipophilic substituent reduces activity in direct relationship to its size.

While there are many similarities in nuclear and serum protein-binding requirements, there are also some significant differences. The major differences occur with regard to the 3′,4′,5′-substituents. As can be noted in Table 3.8, the nuclear receptors preferentially bind to 3′-substituted (distally oriented) compounds, while TBG has maximal binding for 3′,5′-disubstituted compounds with electron-withdrawing groups. Also, from pH dependencies of T_3 and T_4 binding, it appears that the 4′-OH is binding to nuclear receptors in its un-ionized form while TBG data suggest it is the 4′-phenoxide ion that binds (Dietrich et al. 1977). These results agree with the crystallographic observations of T_4 structures in their phenoxide form and T_3 structures as un-ionized hydroxyls.

II. Binding and Potency of TBG

The more recent studies of thyroxine analogue binding to TBG (Snyder et al. 1976) show that all of the structural features of thyroxine are important for optimal binding. The large differences in binding of T_4 versus T_3 compounds reflect the stringent requirement for both the 3′ and 5′ positions to be occupied by electron-withdrawing groups. The unexpectedly high binding affinity of T_3 [previous studies (Hao and Tabachnick 1971; Tabachnik and Korcek, 1978) found little or no binding] indicates that the increased polarization and ionization of the 4′-OH and the hydrophobic interactions of these outer ring iodines are of major importance to TBG binding. These conditions are of almost no importance in nuclear binding (Table 3.8) since T_4 and rT_3 show very little binding affinity and possess little or no biologic potency. It is also apparent from these data that the steric conformation of the alanine side chain, with the presence of both amino and carboxyl groups, is of major importance since modification of this portion of the molecule dramatically decreases the binding affinity.

The great difference between L- versus D-compounds indicates that the stereochemistry of the amino acid plays a significant role in controlling binding. If one assumes that T_4 has two fixed points of attachment to the receptor site, then, as shown in Fig. 3.33, the stereochemical differences between the L- and D-isomers become the relative disposition of the remaining functional groups at the asymmetric α-carbon. Thus, if a specific stereochemical relationship must be maintained between functional groups (NH_3^+ versus COO^-), this disposition can

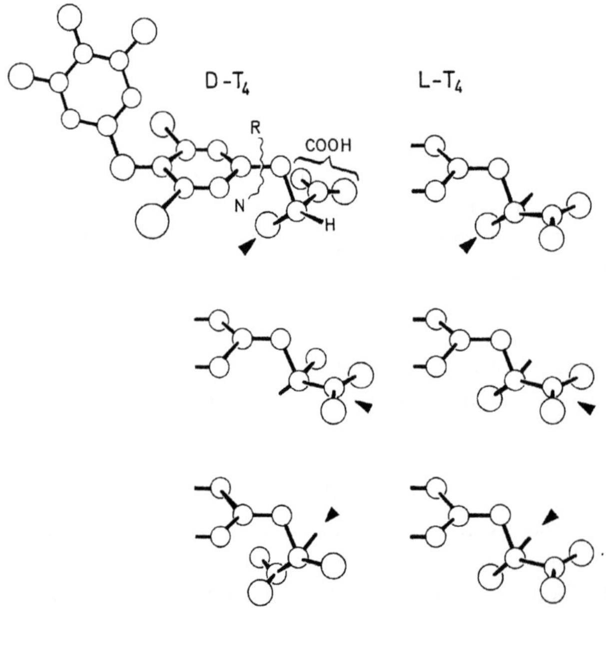

Fig. 3.33. Stereochemical differences between L- and D-isomers of thyronine derivatives. Figure shows spatial orientation of each of the functional groups of the C-alpha carbon (R, N, COOH, H) if the ring and one other functional group are held fixed, respectively. (Cody 1978 a)

only be maintained in one isomer. Therefore, if the amino function must be extended with respect to the ring (i. e., $\chi^1 = 180°$), the carboxylic group has a fixed orientation. It then appears that there is an optimum relative positioning of the amino and carboxylic group that can only be achieved in the L-isomer (Cody 1978 a).

The relative binding affinities for the side chain group follow a linear progression (Table 3.8) with respect to the length (L-alanine > *N*-acetyl > propionic > acetic) where the data of Hao and Tabachnik (1971) show an anomalous ordering (acetic ≫ propionic). Since thyropropionic acid structures have fully extended side chains (i. e., $\chi^1 = -60°$ for T_4), this may be considered the optimum orientation for TBG binding. This conformation is illustrated in Fig. 3.34 which shows optimum overlap between iodothyronine and thyropropionic acid structures.

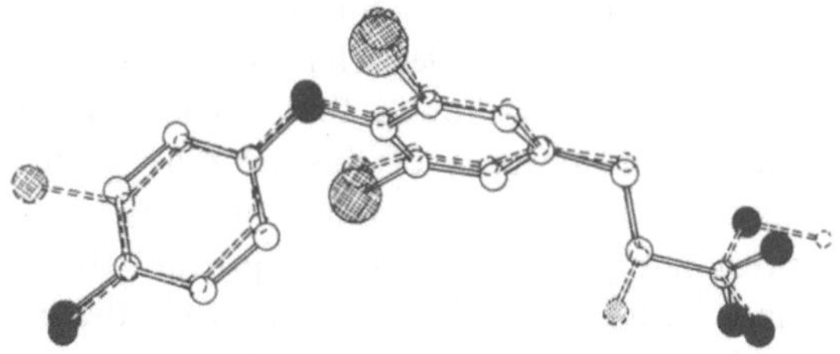

Fig. 3.34. Superimposition of thyropropionic acid (TO12, Table 3.1) on a thyroid hormone (TO03, Table 3.1) (*dotted* figure) showing the complementarity between side chain groups

Considering the fact that the acetic acid analogues have shortened the carbon chain in addition to losing the amino function, one might expect even greater differences in thyropropionic and thyroacetic acid binding affinities. Figure 3.35 shows the superimposition of an observed thyroacetic acid structure with that of an iodothyronine. As can be seen, structurally, one of the acetic acid oxygens can spatially overlap that of the amine. Thus, in an appropriate orientation, these two functional groups could occupy the same environment. Since they are electronically different, this might indicate that their binding environment could accept either group. It was proposed (Hao and Tabachnik 1971) that a histidine group would satisfy these requirements, and thus it is the availability of a charged species that is important to this environment.

Aliphatic substitution in the 1-position is probably critical, both in terms of binding at the receptor site and contributing toward pharmacodynamic properties such as movement through membranes and transport properties, particularly since L-isomers are more potent than the D-isomers (Murray 1974). These side chain effects are apparently intrinsic and not caused by effects of the side chain on the ring system.

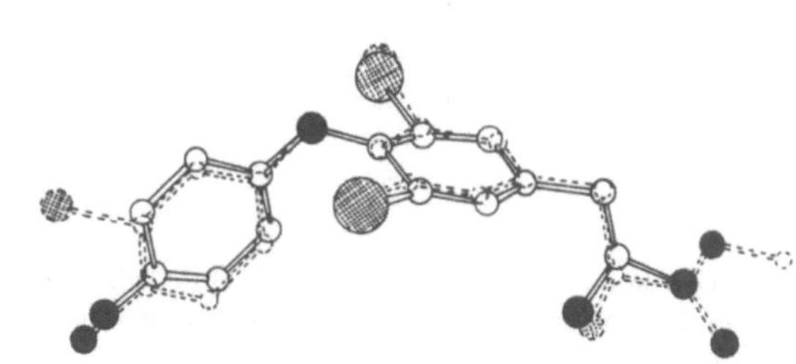

Fig. 3.35. Superimposition of thyroacetic acid (TO11, Table 3.1) on a thyroid hormone (TO03, Table 3.1) (*dotted* figure) showing the spatial complementarity of the side chain functional groups. (Cody 1978 a)

From these TBG binding affinity studies (Snyder et al. 1976) the relative importance of the iodine positions vis-a-vis conformational rigidity can be inferred. It can be seen (Table 3.8) that of primary importance is the 3′,5′-iodines' effect on the pKa of 4′-OH, as well as their hydrophobic interactions. This is reflected in the tighter binding of rT_3 with respect to that of T_3. Also, the ability to maintain a fixed conformation may not be of great importance since rT_3 is not conformationally locked as is T_3. However, this is not to say that the actual binding conformation may not be skewed.

At this point there is a trade-off in the requirement for halogens in both rings as opposed to two halogens in the outer ring since the binding order is 3′,3-T_2 > 3′,5′-T_2 > 3,5-T_2. The latter has a fixed diphenyl ether conformation whereas the former does not. However, it is apparently more important to have at least one inner ring halogen because 3-T_1 binds better than 3′-T_1.

The binding requirements are completely reversed in regard to nuclear receptors and hormone potencies. Here, it is a 3′-substituted compound, conformationally fixed and distally-skewed, that is of key importance. As can be noted by the greater binding and potency of 3′-isopropyl-T_2, the outer ring need not be restricted to electron-withdrawing groups. From these data it is shown that a 3′-substituent (presumably distal) is more important than conformational rigidity since 3,3′-T_2 binds better than 3,5-T_2. Again, while there is no requirement for conformational rigidity in 3,3′-T_2, a skewed diphenyl ether conformation at the binding site is not precluded in any way. The fact that reverse T_3 is the least effective in binding and potency suggests that the negative effects of the 5′-iodine override the loss of conformational rigidity. From this discussion it can be inferred that rT_3 lacks hormonal potency and nuclear binding efficiency on three counts: (1) the formation of a 4′-phenoxide as induced by the 3′,5′-iodine influence on 4′-OH acidity, (2) the bulky 5′-iodine blocking the receptor pocket, and (3) the diphenyl ether is no longer conformationally restricted to be skewed.

The observation that 3′-isopropyl-3,5-diiodothyronine is a more effective protein binder and has greater hormonal potency than T_3 is an enigma. As seen in Fig. 3.36, conformationally 3′-isopropyl T_3 and T_3 (TO07, TO10) (Table 3.1) are similar. Also,

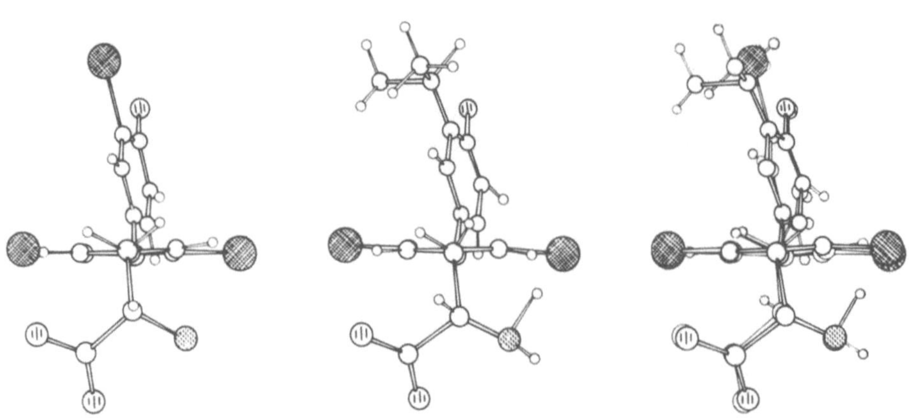

a b c

Fig. 3.36 a–c. Comparison of (**a**) T_3 (TO07, Table 3.1) with (**b**) 3′-isopropyl-T_2 (TO10, Table 3.1), and (**c**) the superimposition of the two to illustrate the relative size of the iodine and isopropyl groups

the volume occupied by the isopropyl group is about equal to that of iodine (Fig. 3.36). Therefore, the two can fit easily into the same receptor site. It may be that the receptor pocket of the 3′-substituent is enhanced by an electron-withdrawing group of this specific size. Aliphatic functional groups larger or smaller than isopropyl do not elicit this same response and are less potent than T_3.

III. Thyroxine-Binding Prealbumin Interactions

Thyroxine-binding prealbumin, which transports both T_4 and the retinol-binding protein for vitamin A, is the first serum protein to have its structure fully defined by chemical and physical studies (Kanda et al. 1974; Blake et al. 1974). X-Ray diffraction studies show it to be a tetrameric protein with a mol. wt. of 54 000 and to have a channel running the length of the molecule.

Low resolution X-ray crystallographic analysis of TBPA complexed with T_4 and T_3 shows that the hormones are bound exclusively to two symmetry-related sites buried deeply within the central channel (Blake and Oatley 1977). Analysis of the free space around the axis of the channel shows that there is a cylindrical hole along the length of the axis about 8 Å in diameter, except at two symmetrically related positions some 4 Å on either side of the center of the channel where the close approach of the side chains causes a local constriction. However, because the thyroid hormones cannot be accommodated by the symmetry requirements of the protein, their exact orientation in the receptor site cannot be defined. Instead, an average position of two symmetry-related orientations is observed.

According to Blake and Oatley (1977) each of the outer ring iodines lies between and in contact with the side-chains of leucines 17 and 110, and each of the inner ring iodines fits into a pocket lined with the methyl groups of threonine 106, alanine 108 and valine 121, and the β- and γ-methylenes of lysine 15. This model also shows that the 4′-OH of T_4 hydrogen bonds, via a water molecule, with the hydroxyls of the serine 117 and threonine 119. The carboxylic acid group of thyroxine interacts with lysine 15 while the amino group interacts with glutamic acid 54. A model of T_4 in this binding site is illustrated in Fig. 3.37. The interaction of T_4 with lysine 15 is further supported by affinity labeling experiments on prealbumin using dansyl chloride (Cheng et al. 1975 and 1977), both of which have been covalently attached to lysine 15.

With this detailed description and knowledge of the structural features of TBPA, combined with the relative binding affinities of thyroid hormone analogues (Table 3.9) to this protein (Andrea 1977), a relatively detailed picture of the hormone–receptor interaction can now be formulated. The most striking feature of these data is that the acid side chain analogues have higher binding affinities than T_4. This is in contrast to the binding order both to the serum protein TBG and the nuclear proteins (Table 3.8). This suggests that the tetra-substituted diphenyl ether nucleus is the key function required for binding. Also, the relative ordering of the 3′,5′-substituted compounds suggests that the hydrophobic interactions of the outer ring are more important than those of the inner ring. TBPA prefers to bind a 4′-phenoxide rather than its un-ionized hydroxyl (Andrea 1977). This is consistent with the crystallographic observations of T_4 structures.

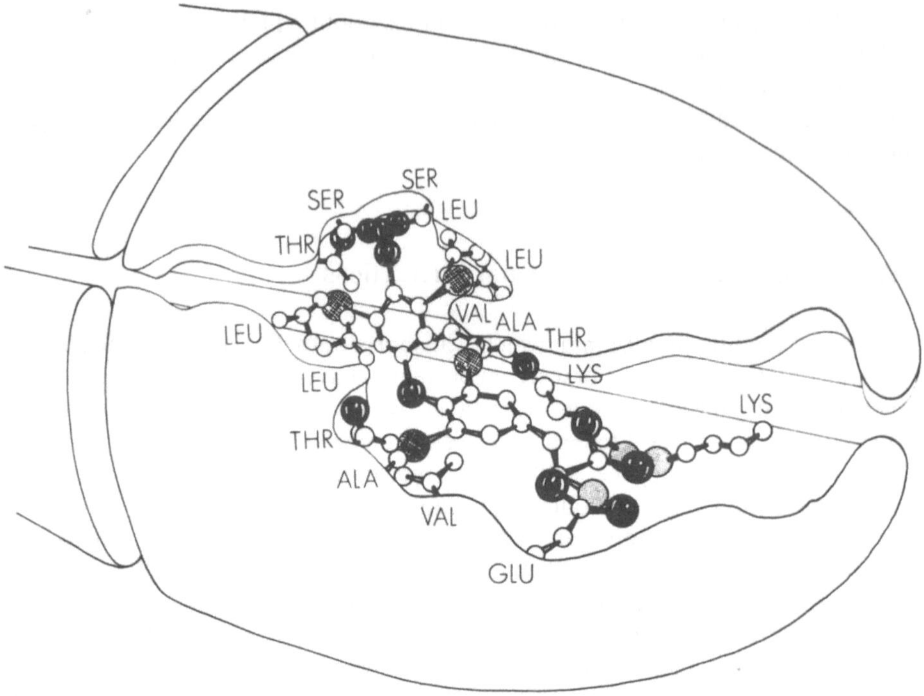

Fig. 3.37. Model representation of T_4–TBPA receptor site based on the results of Blake and Oatley (1977). (Cody 1978 a). The abbreviations are amino acids which come in contact with T_4 at the binding site

Table 3.9. Relative binding affinities of thyroid hormones and analogues for thyroxine binding prealbumin (Andrea 1977, p. 181)

Compound	Binding affinity
Tetraiodothyroacetic acid	100.0%
Tetraiodothyroformic acid	90.2
Tetraiodothyropropionic acid	76.4
Tetraiodothyrobutyric acid	47.6
L-Thyroxine	39.3
Triiodothyroacetic acid	4.7
L-3',5',3-Triiodothyronine	3.1
L-3,5,3'-Triiodothyronine	1.4
D-Thyroxine	0.95
3',5'-DL-Diiodothyronine	0.87
3,3'-L-Diiodothyronine	0.35
Thyroxamine	0.08
D-3,5,3'-Triiodothyronine	0.06
L-3,5-Diiodothyronine	0.03
3'-DL-Iodothyronine	0.01
3-L-Iodothyronine	<0.01
Thyronine	<0.01

In an attempt to explain the relative ordering of the side chain analogues and the disparate binding differences between L- and D-isomers, the binding free energies of the various analogues in the presence of the charged side chain groups of the TBPA binding cavity were computed (Andrea 1977; Andrea et al. 1978). These data were interpreted to indicate that the side chain of T_4P, L-T_4, D-T_4, and T_4NH_3 has a net two attractive, zero, zero, and two repulsive interactions respectively, with the TBPA groups in their immediate vicinity. The relative ordering of the side chain analogues ($T_4A > T_4F > T_4P > T_4B$) was viewed (Andrea 1977) as an indication that the analogues are anchored deep within the binding channel with the carboxylic groups experiencing a net attraction from lysine 15.

The most striking feature of the data listed in Table 3.9 is that the acid metabolites bind more strongly to TBPA than T_4; this feature is directly opposite to that of the order observed for TBG and the nuclear proteins. A factor that may influence these parameters is the relative importance to binding of the diphenyl ether conformation and the side chain conformation. As has been observed (Cody et al. 1977b), thyroactive acid structures prefer a skewed conformation whereas the full amino acid structures prefer a twist-skewed conformation. As illustrated in Fig. 3.17, there is a significant displacement in the 4′-OH position between these two conformers. If, as proposed, the tetraiododiphenyl ether portion of the molecule is tightly bound deeply within the channel and forms a specific hydrogen bond through the 4′-phenoxide to a water (Blake and Oatley 1977) or some other peptide functional group, then the 4′-phenoxy ring would have a primary influence on binding. Therefore, if 4′-phenoxy interactions control binding, these differences will affect the position of the side chain groups within the binding channel. The binding volume described by the thyroactive acid structures is illustrated in Fig. 3.38, which also shows the effective volume taken up by T_4 when its 4′-phenoxide is bound in a twist-skewed position.

When the molecular structure of the acid metabolite T_4A (dark, Fig. 3.38) is successively superimposed over that of (a) T_4F, (b) T_4P, (c) T_4, and (d) all of them; it can be seen that the acid side chains describe a probable binding volume from which the T_4 amine is excluded. In addition, the T_4 inner ring has the largest deviation from the positional range described by the acid metabolites. Also, the carboxylic oxygens of the various metabolites (except T_4F), irrespective of composition, tend to cluster together, suggesting that this feature may also be of importance in determining relative binding affinity. However, because of the T_4 orientation disorder in the protein complex, this structural model is not a sensitive measure of the observed correlations between diphenyl ether conformations and binding affinity data.

The differences in binding orders between TBPA and TBG suggest that different structural features may play a key role in receptor interactions. It has been shown that TBG also preferentially binds to a tetraiodo-4′-phenoxide ion, but since T_4 is the strongest binder, this suggests a different side chain sterechemistry. Here we can assume that it is the twist-skewed diphenyl ether conformation that orients the T_4 side chain for optimal receptor–hormone interactions. In the case of the nuclear proteins optimal binding is observed for a distally oriented 3′-I and a 4′-hydroxyl. Side chain requirements appear to be similar to those of TBG.

Therefore, changes in the relative binding affinities of thyroid hormone structures to receptors will ultimately depend on the specific steric requirements of the binding

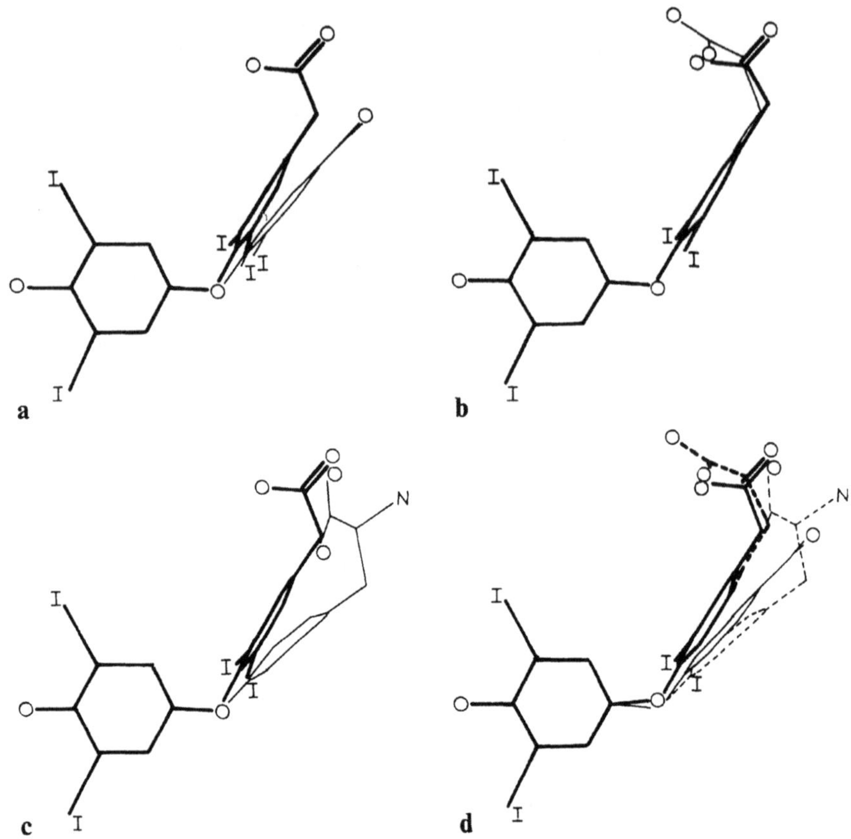

Fig. 3.38 a–d. Structural consequence of skewed versus twist-skewed diphenyl ether conformation assuming a fixed orientation of the outer phenyl ring: **a** T_4A (*dark*) superimposed on T_4F [TO04, TO15, Table 3.1]; **b** T_4A (*dark*) superimposed on T_4P [TO04, TO19]; **c** T_4A (*dark*) superimposed on T_4 [TO04, TO16A2]; **d** all four structures superimposed

site and the ability of the hormones to adopt the required conformation. In addition, the net charge of the hormone could also influence its binding ability. Thus, the observation of conformational patterns among thyroactive structures which correlate with function, activity, and binding data provide useful information in describing specific types of hormone–receptor interactions.

F. Summary

The comprehensive analysis of three-dimensional structures of the thyroid hormones and their analogues has provided a concise description of the molecular conformation of these hormones. The observation of patterns of conformational isomerism (Cody 1978 a) in these structures suggests that, while these hormones have flexibility (i. e., rotation about single bonds with limited steric hindrance), certain "conformational families" or small sets of families peculiar to each group of molecules (e. g., acids versus amino acids) exist and are favored for a particular type of hormone–receptor interaction. A family of conformations is then a relatively small group of structures related to one another by minor changes in rotation angles (Williams 1977). Thus, the conformational families observed in thyroid hormone structures that could play important roles in protein hormone interactions include (1) skewed/twist-skewed diphenyl ether conformation, (2) distal/proximal 3′-orientation, and (3) cisoid/transiod overall conformation.

Protein–hormone binding is, in essence, an interaction between a biologic macromolecule and a small molecule. This type of complexation is only one of many different types of protein interactions, all of which are molecularly intertwined in a cellular environment (Klotz, 1973). When a semirigid hormone such as T_4 binds to a mobile receptor (protein, membrane, etc.), the shape and function of both can change (Williams 1977). Thus, the study of the nature and extent of these changes by several independent methods provides an insight into the mode of action of these hormones. Furthermore, whether a molecule binds or not depends on whether it can reach a certain site. Therefore, knowledge of the molecular dynamics of hormone–receptor interactions is important because small molecule binding can play a crucial role in this dynamic process which then can lead to the initiation of a hormonal response.

While these X-ray crystallographic studies provide a static picture of the hormone in various states, data on substrate conformational flexibility are vital to the accurate interpretation of molecular details at the active site. When the crystal structures of thyroid hormone binding proteins are determined, the static matching of hormone to receptor site could play an important role in the interpretation of dynamic processes of hormone binding and action. Thus, these studies on the interaction of the thyroid hormones with various kinds of sites, including receptor sites in transport systems, membranes, or enzymes, have provided valuable clues to the mechanisms by which these hormones can exert their pharmacologic and therapeutic effects.

In conclusion, these crystallographic data have shown: (1) the solid state observation of both distal and proximal 3′-iodine orientations, (2) a skewed or twist-skewed diphenyl ether conformation, (3) a cisoid or transoid overall conformation, (4) long-range conformational transmission from side chain substituent influence, (5) correlations of outer phenyl ring geometry with 4′-OH acidity and degree of ionization, (6) intermolecular charge-transfer interactions, (7) hydrogen bond directionality consistent with protein binding requirements conformations to plasma and nuclear proteins.

It is hoped that these data will provide a better understanding of the basic molecular mechanisms of thyroid hormone action and will prove to be a key to a fuller interpretation of extant biochemical studies of thyroid hormones.

Acknowledgments. These studies were supported in part by United States Health Service Grant AM-15051. Graphs and tables were prepared through interrogation of the thyroid data stored in the National Institutes of Health PROPHET system, an NIH interactive computer network. The author wishes to express her appreciation to Dr. Jane Griffin for valuable discussion of the material presented in this manuscript. The technical and secretarial assistance of Dr. John Hazel, Miss Gloria Del Bel, Miss Telda Tugac, Mrs. Catherine DeVine, Mrs. Brenda Giacchi, Miss Kathleen Castiglione, and Mrs. Estelle Robel are gratefully acknowledged.

Chapter 4

Concentration of Triiodothyronines (T_3 and Reverse T_3) in Serum and Other Body Fluids

The availability of sensitive, rapid, and precise methods for the measurement of T_3 and rT_3 has been a key factor responsible for the recent major improvements in our understanding of thyroid hormone physiology. This chapter reviews some methods of measurement and data regarding T_3 concentrations in the serum and/or amniotic fluid of healthy individuals, those with thyroid disease, and in those with nonthyroidal systemic diseases. The data on serum T_4 levels are also described when considered relevant to the understanding of the nature and/or the basis of the changes in the levels of circulating thyroid hormone levels in various circumstances.

A. Methods of Measurement

I. T_3 (3,5,3′-T_3)

Following the discovery of T_3 in human serum in 1952, the assessment of its concentration was the next logical step, which led to understanding of its importance in the thyroid hormone economy. The initial approach to serum T_3 measurements consisted of extraction of iodothyronines from serum, separation of T_3 from T_4 by paper chromatography, and quantitation of T_3 iodine (T_3I) by chemical means. Pind (1957) estimated that the serum concentration of T_3I in euthyroid subjects averages 150 ng/dl. Since T_3 is comprised of 57% iodine by weight, Pind's estimates corresponded to a mean serum-T_3 concentration of 257 ng/dl. Employing a method similar in principle to that of Pind, Maclagan et al. (1957) found normal serum T_3 concentration to be 500 ng/dl or less in euthyroid individuals and between 1000 and 4000 ng/dl in hyperthyroid patients. However, the detection threshold of this method was very high and the technique is tedious as well as time consuming. Therefore, it was not applied to routine measurements of T_3 in the diagnosis of thyroid disease.

A major improvement in T_3 methodology was brought about by Naumann et al. in 1967. They obtained T_3 and T_4 from serum by a methanol–chloroform extraction, separated T_3 from T_4 by paper chromatography, and adapted a modification of Murphy-Pattee's CPBA for quantitation of T_3 in T_3 zones of chromatograms. Using this approach, they reported a mean normal serum T_3 concentration of 330 ng/dl. However, Sterling and co-workers (1969) soon critized Naumann et al. for their method of T_3 measurement because it yielded spuriously high values on account of the formation of methyl ester of T_4 during methanol–chloroform extraction of serum. They noted that in all of the usual chromatographic systems, T_4 methyl ester migrates into or very close to T_3 zones on the chromatograms and that its inclusion in T_3 eluates results in artifactually high estimates of T_3 measured by CPBA in the final step. Sterling et al. (1969) circumvented the problem of formation of alcohol esters of T_4 by using a column of an ion exchange resin (Dowex AG-50 W-X_2, H+ form, 100-200 mesh, Bio Rad Laboratories, Richmond, California) for extraction of T_3 and T_4 from serum. They also used paper chromatography to separate T_3 from T_4, followed by a modification of Murphy-Pattee's CPBA for final quantitation of T_3 in T_3 zones of the chromatograms. The mean normal serum T_3 concentration by the method of Sterling et al. (1969) approximated 220 ng/dl.

Although the method of Sterling et al. (1969) clearly provided important information on the physiologic significance of T_3, it was quite tedious and time consuming and, in most instances, required relatively large volumes (~5 ml) of serum for T_3 measurements. Moreover, studies from several laboratories, notably those of Larsen (1971, 1972 b, c) and Fisher and Dussault (1971) provided evidence suggesting that the method of Sterling et al. yielded falsely high measurements just as did the technique of Naumann et al. This seemed so because of two apparent complications during the available chromatographic methods for separation of T_3 to T_4: (1) contamination of T_3 by some T_4, and (2) artifactual deiodination of T_4 to T_3. Studies of Benotti and co-workers (1970) suggested that T_3 isolated by paper chromatography of serum extracts may be contaminated with about 0.5% of T_4. Since T_4 may cause 2.5 times or greater displacement of radioactive T_3 from TBG in CPBA than an equal weight of T_4, contamination of 0.5% of normal T_4 (4–11 µg/dl) appeared to artifactually increase serum T_3 concentration estimates by 50 to 138 ng/dl. Moreover, it was estimated that some 0.3%–0.4% of T_4 may be monodeiodinated to T_3 during chromatography for separation of T_3 from T_4; this seemingly minor problem caused an artifactual increase of 12 to 44 ng/dl in the estimates of serum T_3 by the Sterling method. Concern over these various matters led Dussault et al. (1971) to develop and carefully evaluate a double column chromatography method for the measurement of T_3. They observed that, when corrected for methodologic artifacts, the range of serum T_3 concentration in normal subjects lies between 25 and 203 ng/dl (mean, ±SD, 98±38). However, like other methods then available, the method of Dussault et al. (1971) for T_3 measurement was time consuming and cumbersome. In addition, large corrections for methodologic artifacts were a serious problem.

Brown et al. (1970) first reported success in producing a T_3-binding antiserum in rabbits immunized with conjugates of T_3 with succinylate polylysine. This finding represented an important accomplishment because iodothyronines had generally been considered nonantigenic. Anti-T_3 produced by Brown et al. (1970) was, however, not adequate; T_4 had a cross-reaction of about 5% with T_3-binding sites on this antiserum. Therefore, for appropriate measurements of T_3 in serum, Brown et al. (1971) found it necessary to employ extraction and chromatography steps similar to those used by Sterling et al. (1969) before using anti-T_3 antibody in RIA chromatographic T_3 zone eluates. Using the RIA, Ekins (in Sterling K. 1970) first reported an intriguing finding that T_3 may normally be undetectable (< 10 ng/dl) in human serum. However, subsequent, more detailed studies of Ekins and co-workers yielded results of normal serum T_3 concentration between 75–160 ng/dl (mean ≃120) (Brown et al. 1971). Soon after the report by Brown and co-workers on the production of T_3-binding antibodies, highly specific anti-T_3 antibodies were generated by at least two other groups. Chopra et al. (1971 b, c) reported a finding of T_3-binding antibodies by immunization of rabbits with human thyroglobulin, and Gharib et al. (1970, 1971) obtained T_3-binding antibodies by immunizing rabbits with human serum albumin (HSA-T_3) conjugates.

Both groups applied T_3 antibodies in an RIA of unextracted serum but with markedly different results. Chopra et al. (1971 b) observed normal serum T_3 to range between <100 and 170 ng/dl, whereas Gharib et al. noted mean (±S.D.) normal serum T_3 concentration to be 218±55 ng/100 ml. The difference may have been related to a variation in the control of the interference of the T_3-binding serum proteins in T_3 RIA. T_3-binding proteins (e.g., TBG) complicate T_3 measurements with RIA of unextracted serum by (1) limiting the availability of T_3 for reaction with the antibody and (2) competing with the antibody for radioactive T_3 used as the ligand. Chopra et al. had added an equal excess of nonradioactive T_4 to all standards and unknowns to displace T_3 bound to serum proteins (thereby rendering it available for measurement in RIA) and to minimize the binding of radioactive (or nonradioactive) T_3 to serum proteins. Gharib et al. had used merthiolate in their RIA incubation mixture, but its purpose or adequacy to block interference of serum proteins was not stated clearly. In any case, the results of Gharib et al. with serum T_3 concentration supported the accuracy of serum T_3 values measured by the method of Sterling et al. (1969) and thereby served to perpetuate (actually enhance) the then prevalent controversy concerning the accurate level of T_3 in normal man.

Shortly thereafter, several other investigators were successful in producing T_3-binding antibodies in rabbits by immunizing patients with conjugates of T_3 in bovine serum albumin (BSA), polyglutamic acid, or polylysine (Table 4.1). Several different agents, including tetrachlorthyronine, diphenylhydantoin sodium (Dilantin), sodium salicylate, and 8-anilino-1-naphthalene sulfonic acid, were employed in whole serum RIAs of T_3 to block the interference caused by T_3-binding proteins in serum. These procedures yielded the estimates of normal serum T_3 concentration in the range of 50–210 ng/dl with mean values varying between 110 and 145 ng/dl. These relatively modest variations in mean normal serum T_3 were observed despite the use of (1) varying sources of proteins, e.g., 5% HSA, hypothyroid sheep serum, or activated charcoal-treated (T_3 and T_4 free) human serum, in the standards to render them comparable to the unknown test sera, and (2) different methods of separation of radioactive T_3 bound to the antibody from unbound radioactivity, including "second" antibody, dextran-coated charcoal, ammonium sulfate precipitation, or polyethylene glycol precipitation. Other investigators, apparently unconvinced of the accuracy of the simple whole serum RIAs devised somewhat more cumbersome methods of RIA sera extracts (Surks et al. 1972; Patel et al. 1973 a), but results were not significantly different from those with whole serum RIAs. However, another modification of T_3 RIA, which involved inactivation of TBG by heating the serum at 56°C for 1 h prior to immunoassay, yielded 189 ng/dl as the mean value for normal serum T_3 concentration. The reasons for this high value compared with that obtained by other RIAs are not known. Some monodeiodination of T_4 to T_3 in vitro and incomplete inactivation of TBG during heat treatment of serum are possibilities. Alternatively, the various other RIAs may underestimate serum T_3 concentration.

In addition to chemical and radioassay mathods, serum T_3 concentration has also been measured by gas–liquid chromatography and by double isotope

Table 4.1. Relative cross-reactivity[a] of thyroid hormone derivatives with some T_3-binding antisera

	1	2	3	4	5
Compound	Brown[b] et al. 1971	Gharib et al. 1971	Chopra et al. 1972a	Lieblich and Utiger 1972	Burger et al. 1975
D-T_3	–	39	140	82	–
3,5,3′-Triiodothyropropionic acid	–	36	129	53	–
3,5,3′-Triiodothyroacetic acid	~30	35	40	32	–
3,3′,5′-T_3 (rT_3)	–	–	< 0.1	–	–
Reverse triiodothyropropionic	–	< 0.01	–	–	–
L-T_4	2–5	0.33	0.05	0.10 or less	0.30
D-T_4	2–5	< 0.1	0.2	0.16	–
Tetraiodothyroacetic acid	< 0.1	0.04	0.8	0.16	–
Tetraiodothyropropionic acid	< 0.1	< 0.1	–	0.36	–
3,5-L-Diiodothyronine (3,5-T_2)	–	1.4	0.6	0.09	–
3,3′-T_2	–	5.0	3.0	–	–
3,3′-Diiodothyropropionic acid	–	0.3	–	–	–
Thyronine	–	< 0.01	–	< 0.001	–
Diiodotyrosine	< 0.1	< 0.01	< 0.001	< 0.001	–
Monoiodotyrosine	< 0.1	< 0.01	< 0.001	< 0.001	–
Iodine	–	< 0.001	< 0.001	–	–

[a] Relative reactivity (an arbitrary value if L-T_3 = 100).
[b] Antibodies were produced by immunization with conjugates of T_3 with poly-L-lysine in column 1; HSA in 2; thyroglobulin in 3; BSA in 4, and hemocyanin in 5. Carbodiimide was used for conjugation in 1–4 and diazotized benzidine in 5.

derivative methods. Both of these techniques are tedious and require more specialized instrumentation than for RIAs. Using gas chromatography, Hollander (1968) initially estimated the normal serum T_3 concentration to be as high as 450 ng/dl. However, subsequent studies indicated errors in these measurements. Hollander and co-workers later found normal serum T_3 concentration to approximate 137 ng/dl whether measured by gas–liquid chromatography or RIA of unextracted serum (Nihei et al. 1971). In the only report of serum T_3 measurement by a double isotope derivative method, the mean value was 226 ng/dl (Hagen et al. 1970, 1973). Why this is so much higher than that measured by most RIAs is not known and experience with this method has remained very limited.

It is obvious that, despite many years of intensive investigation using various innovative techniques by several groups in different countries, the absolute "true" range and mean values of serum T_3 concentration in normal man remain undetermined. Fortunately, however, investigators have not let this circumstance deter them from investigating the significance of T_3 in thyroid hormone economy. Through the use of apparently valid and accurate (but probably only semivalid and semiaccurate) techniques, a great deal of interesting information has been gathered regarding alterations in serum T_3 in various physiologic states and in thyroid disease. RIA has been the tool used most frequently in these investigations. An RIA of T_3 on unextracted serum is a relatively simple, precise, and quick method, which makes it feasible to examine a large number of test samples simultaneously. The results obtained, although only approximate in "absolute" terms yield accurate relative information in various disease states. The description that follows is an RIA system used by the author. It is hoped that this information will assist those attempting to put together an RIA of T_3 for their own use.

1. T_3 Radioimmunoassay

a) Reagents

T_3-Binding antiserum. Antiserum suitable for RIA of T_3 may be produced by immunization of rabbits with T_3 conjugated with thyroglobulin, hemocyanin, HSA, or BSA.

A convenient protocol for conjugation adapted from the method of Oliver et al. (1968) is as follows: To 50 mg protein (thyroglobulin, HSA, or BSA) in 25 ml of phosphate buffer saline (PBS) (0.01 *M* phosphate, 0.14 *M* NaCl, pH 7.4) add, while stirring, 20 mg T_3 dissolved in 4 ml dimethyl-foramide and 30 mg 1-cyclo-hexyl-3 (2-morpholinoethyl) carbodiimide metho-*p*-toluene-sulfonate (Morpho-CDI, Aldrich Chemical Co., Inc., Milwaukee, Wis.). After 10 min, add an additional 10 mg Morpho-CDI. Keep stirring the solution at room temperature in the dark for 18 h. Dialyze the reaction mixture against three changes of PBS each time, using 4 liters for 24 h at 4 °C. The solution containing the conjugate may then be stored frozen at −10 °C. An emulsion of equal volumes of solution of the conjugate containing about 1 mg of conjugated protein and complete Freund's adjuvant may be used to immunize New Zealand rabbits in multiple sites at 1–3 week intervals for six to eight injections. Rabbit sera are obtained at 10 days after the last injection and an optimal serum dilution for RIA is determined. An antiserum dilution which binds 30%–50% of a tracer amount ($\simeq 0.1$ ng) of radioactive (^{125}I)-T_3 to antibody is usually used; in the experience of various investigators, the titers of T_3-binding antisera have varied from 1/250 to 1/100,000; low titer of the antiserum does not necessarily imply low-affinity antisera.

Immunization of rabbits with human thyroglobulin alone also leads to the generation of T_3-binding antibodies (Chopra et al. 1971 b, c). This is so because thyroglobulin harbors T_3 (and T_4) in a natural covalent linkage. Interestingly, sera of rabbits immunized with thyroglobulin contain antibodies that bind T_3 as well as T_4 relatively specifically; T_4 cross-reacts minimally with T_3 binding sites on the immunized rabbit immunoglobulin, and vice versa. Thus, sera of rabbits immunized with thyroglobulin can yield antibody reagents useful for RIAs of both T_3 and T_4. While this is clearly a convenient and practical source of anti-T_4 antibodies, the titer of T_3-binding antibodies so produced is usually low. Therefore, anti-T_3 antibodies have been generally produced by using conjugates of T_3 as antigens with one or another of several proteins.

Since T_3 is present in a very small quantity in the blood (about 1/70th that of T_4), it is necessary to use a T_3-binding antiserum in the RIA that is very specific and that allows detection of pg quantities of nonradioactive T_3. An antiserum that permits detection of 50 pg or less of nonradioactive T_3 should be suitable for T_3 RIA.

Specificity of the antiserum may be assessed by studying the inhibition of the binding of radioactive T_3 by the antiserum with two or more concentrations of a variety of substances; examples of specificity of some antisera that have been found satisfactory for T_3 RIAs are presented in Table 4.2. It may be recalled that

Table 4.2. Estimates of serum T_3 concentrations as measured by various methods

Method		Reference	Serum T_3 concentration (ng/100 ml)		
			Euthyroid	Hyperthyroid	Hypothyroid
I.	Extraction, paper chromatography, chemical measurement of iodine in T_3 zone	Pind 1957	257± 68	–	–
		Maclagan et al. 1957	up to 500	1000–4000	<500
II.	Extraction, gas (or gas–liquid) chromatography	Hollander, 1968	450±100	1210± 420	200± 50
		Nihei et al. 1971	137± 23	510± 131	68± 12
III. (a)	Extraction with organic solvents, paper chromatography, CPBA	Nauman et al. 1967	330± 70	710± 100	100± 30
III. (b)	Improved extraction with organic solvents, paper chromatography CPBA	Sterling et al. 1969	220± 27	752± 282	98± 48
III. (c)	Same as III (b) with some corrections for artifacts of paper chromatography	Larsen 1971	180± 40	670± 330	66± 39
III. (d)	Extraction of iodothyronines and separation of T_3 from T_4 by column chromatography, CPBA and correction for procedural artifacts	Dussault et al. 1971	98± 48	443± 51	<25
IV.	Extraction by anion-exchange resin, paper chromatography, RIA	Brown et al. 1970	75–160	290– 860	–
V.	RIA of unextracted serum but without evidence of adequate control of interference by T_3 binding proteins	Gharib et al. 1970	218± 55	760± 289	103± 43
VI. (a)	RIA of unextracted serum using T_4 as a blocking agent to inhibit interference of T_3 binding proteins in RIA	Chopra et al. 1971b	<100–170	<100–1300	<100

Continued next page

Table 4.2 (continued)

	Method	Reference	Serum T_3 concentration (ng/100 ml)		
			Euthyroid	Hyperthyroid	Hypothyroid
VI. (b)	RIA of unextracted serum using tetra-chlorthyronine in place of T_4 in VI. (a)	Mitsuma et al. 1971	138 ± 23	494 ± 265	62 ± 9
VI. (c)	RIA of unextracted serum using dilantin in place of T_4 in VI. (a)	Lieblich and Utiger, 1972	145 ± 25	429 ± 146	99 ± 24
VI. (d)	RIA of unextracted serum using sodium salicylate in place of T_4 in VI. (a)	Larsen 1972 a	110 ± 25	546 ± 442	39 ± 21
VI. (e)	RIA of unextracted serum using 8-anilino-1-naphthalene sulfonic acid (ANS) in place of T_4 in VI. (a)	Mitsuma et al. 1972	134 ± 24	486 ± 255	67 ± 8
		Chopra et al. 1972 a	113 ± 33	491 ± 232	40 ± 27
VI. (f)	RIA of unextracted serum following heat inactivation of TBG in serum	Sterling and Milch 1974	189 ± 30	838 ± 398	47 ± 39
VII. (a)	RIA of extracts obtained by absorption of serum to sephadex (G25) columns at alkaline pH	Surks, et al. 1972	146 ± 24	665 ± 289	44 ± 26
VII. (b)	Direct RIA of ethanol extracts of sera	Patel et al. 1973 a	87 – 177	176 – 1150	<6 – 137
VIII.	Double isotope derivative technique	Hagen et al. 1973	226 ± 82	897 ± 421	92 ± 51

commercial T_4 preparations were found to be contaminated with T_3 to a variable degree. Therefore, a more complete assessment of the cross-reaction of T_4 may require study after purification of T_4.

Barbital buffer. The buffer contains 0.075 *M* barbital, pH 8.6, with 1% normal rabbit serum and 0.1% sodium azide. Barbital buffer is available commercially in convenient ready-to-use packages. (B-2 buffer, Beckman Inc., Fullerton, California).

T_3-Free serum. We have found that serum from a sheep 6 weeks after total surgical thyroidectomy is a suitable source of T_3-free serum (Chopra et al. 1972 a). Iodothyronine-free serum may also be prepared by the treatment of pooled human serum with Norit A decolorizing pharmaceutical charcoal yielding satisfactory

results (Larsen 1972c). This procedure, in brief, involves the addition of 7.5 g of charcoal per 100 ml of serum, stirring overnight at 4 °C, followed by centrifugation at 25000 $\times g$ for three successive 1-h periods to remove charcoal (Larsen 1972c). Alternatively, following overnight mixing of activated charcoal and serum, charcoal may be removed by passing the serum through a Seitz filter (Grade 53, size 6, Republic Seitz Filter Corp., Milldale, Conn.) using vacuum suction. Thyroid hormone-free serum can also be prepared by use of an ion exchange resin (Chopra 1972).

Radioactive (^{125}I)-T_3. This assay (specific activity 80 μc/μg or higher) may be obtained from Industrial Nuclear Inc., St. Louis, Mo. or Abott Laboratories, North Chicago, Ill.

8-Anilino-1-naphthalene sulfonic acid. This may be obtained from K and K Laboratories, Plainview, NY.

Reagent grade Na-L-T_3. This may be obtained from Mann Research Laboratories or Aldrich Chemical Co., Inc., Milwaukee, Wis. It is dissolved and diluted to a concentration of 10 μg per ml in 0.01 *M* NaOH. Dilutions for use in standard curve, i.e., 0.1–100 ng per ml T_3, are made in barbital buffer, described above.

b) Procedure

The procedure, which has been described in detail elsewhere (Chopra et al. 1972a, Chopra 1972), involves addition of various reagents in 10×75 mm glass tubes placed in an acrylic test tube rack (Crossman Manufacturing Company, Los Angeles, CA) that holds up to 243 tubes. The reagents are added in the following order:

1) Barbital buffer, volume to adjust to a final volume of 1 ml.
2) 200 μl of T_3-free serum in the standards and 200 μl of unknowns in other tubes.
3) ANS, 200 μg (100 μl of a fresh solution containing 2 mg per ml).
4) 100 μl of various concentrations of standards to provide 10 pg to 10 ng T_3 in tubes for standard curve.
5) 100 μl of T_3-binding rabbit antiserum diluted so as to bind about 30%–50% of trace amount of (^{125}I)-T_3 in the absence of added nonradioactive T_3.
6) 100 μl of barbital buffer containing approximately 10000 cpm of (^{125}I)-T_3 (~0.1 ng T_3).

The reagents added to the tubes are mixed by swirling after steps 4, 5, and 6. The tubes are incubated for 24 h at 4 °C. A previously titered goat antirabbit gamma globulin (~50–100 μl) is then added and the tubes are reincubated to allow precipitation of antibody-bound radioactive T_3. The tubes are then centrifuged at 2000 rpm for 30 min, the supernatant is aspirated or decanted, and the radioactivity in the precipitates is determined in a γ-scintillation counter. A convenient decanting mechanism used in the author's laboratory is shown in Fig. 4.1 It is a rubber sheet which has been perforated to accommodate snugly 10×75 mm glass culture tubes used in the RIA. It can be used to decant simultaneously as many as 243 tubes (or even more if larger assay racks are used).

Each assay should include two tubes in which 100 μl of buffer is added instead of T_3-binding antiserum; the counts in the precipitates of these tubes provide an index of radioactivity trapped nonspecifically and should be subtracted from the counts in all tubes. In addition, each assay should include two tubes in which all reagents are added except nonradioactive T_3. It is convenient to assign an arbitrary value of 100% to the precipitate counts in these tubes; the counts in other tubes in the assay can then be expressed as a percent of the counts in zero-T_3 concentration in the

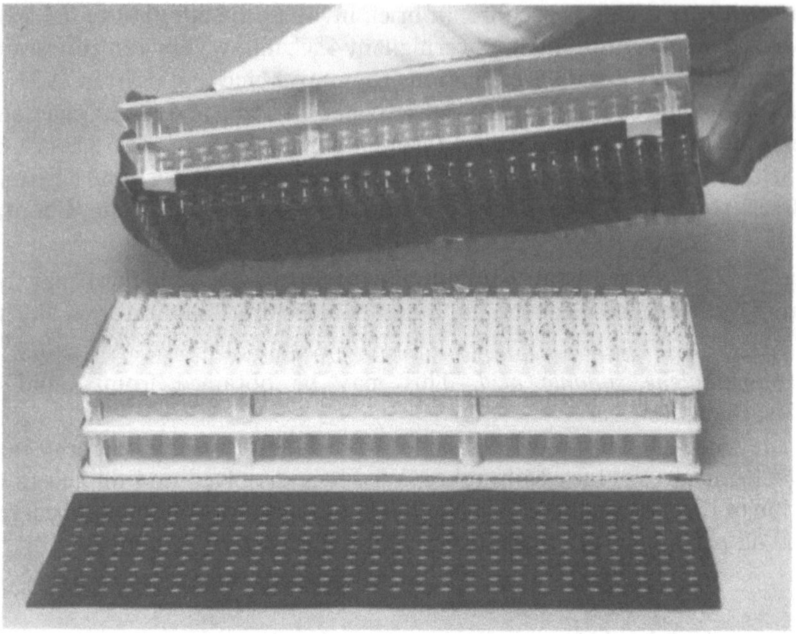

Fig. 4.1. A simple system for decanting supernatants after centrifugation of RIA tubes for separation of bound from free radioactivity. A rubber sheet with perforations to fit the RIA tubes snugly is placed on the assay rack and taped down; the rack is inverted to decant the supernatant. The inverted rack is then placed on absorbent paper to remove any liquid still adhering to the margins of the tubes

standards on the abscissa. Knowing the percent of bound radioactivity in the unknowns, their serum T_3 concentrations can be read directly from the abscissa of the plot.

A disadvantage of the double antibody system for the separation of bound from free radioactive T_3, while convenient and precise, is that the results are not available until the day after the assay. If it is important to obtain results of T_4 estimation on the day of completion of a run, separation of bound from free radioactivity may be accomplished with the use of dextran-coated charcoal, ammonium sulfate or polyethylene glycol (Carbowax 6000). Polyethylene glycol may be used in a final concentration of 12%–15% in order to precipitate immunoglobulin antibodies and the hormone bound to them. Nonspecifically bound (or trapped) radioactivity tends to be higher in RIA systems using charcoal or polyethylene glycol methods than in those using a second antibody for the separation of bound from free radioactivity. One may achieve the advantages of both polyethylene glycol and second antibody methods by combining these reagents for separation of bound from free hormone. For this purpose, the addition of a second antibody is followed by the addition of polyethylene glycol in a final concentration of 3%–4% (cf. 12%–15% mentioned above). Tubes are then incubated at room temperature for 30 min and centrifuged at 1000 $\times g$ at 4 °C for 30 min; the bound radioactivity settles in the precipitate.

Before using the RIA on a routine basis, it is important to examine its validity by studies of recovery, precision, and reproducibility. Some examples of these examinations may be found in original publications of T_3 RIA (e. g., Chopra et al. 1971 b, 1972 a).

II. Reverse T_3 (3,3',5'-T_3, rT_3)

Studies until 1972 had suggested that T_4 is randomly monodeiodinated in extrathyroidal tissues to either T_3 or rT_3. To examine directly the existence and quantitative significance of the pathway of inner-ring monodeiodination of T_4 to rT_3, a method of rT_3 measurement was required. Encouraged by observations on the remarkable specificity of iodothyronine (T_3 and T_4) binding antisera, we undertook preparation of anti-rT_3 antibody in rabbits for an RIA. D,L-Reverse T_3, the only available form of rT_3 at the time, was obtained through the kind courtesy of Dr. Robert Meltzer of Warner Lambert Research Institute, New Jersey. This was conjugated to HSA and used for immunization of rabbits in a manner similar to that described above for T_3. Highly specific rT_3-binding antibody was produced and employed in an RIA of rT_3. Even T_3 that differs from rT_3 only in placement of iodine atoms on the iodothyronine nucleus cross-reacted minimally, less than 0.1%. The cross-reactions of other iodothyronines and their analogues with this anti-rT_3 are shown in Table 4.3.

Table 4.3. Reactivity of various thyroid homone derivatives with rT_3-binding antibodies[a]

	Reference					
	Chopra 1974	Meinhold et al. 1975	Nicod et al. 1976	Ratcliffe et al. 1976		Burman et al. 1977 b
Compound	D,L-rT_3 = 100	D,L-rT_3 = 100	L-rT_3 = 100	D,L-rT_3 = 100	L-rT_3 = 100	L-rT_3 or D,L-rT_3 = 100
L-T_3	0.02[a]	0.02	0.04	<0.003	<0.004	<0.05
D-T_3	0.006	<0.032	–	–	–	<1.0
TRIAC	0.003	–	<0.01	<0.002	<0.01	<0.01
3,5,3'-L-Triiodothyropropionic acid	0.005					
L-T_4	0.06	≤0.1	0.06	0.15	0.14	<0.01
D-T_4	0.045					
TETRAC	0.034		0.02	<0.004	0.010	<0.01
Desaminothyroxine	0.045					
3,5-L-Diiodothyronine	< 0.002		<0.01			
3,3'-L-Diiodothyronine	10.0	1.0	0.6	3.9	0.42	0.1, 1.0[b]
3,5-L-Diiodothyropropionic acid	0.005					
3-L-Monoiodothyronine	0.24					
L-Thyronine	< 0.002					
Diiodotyrosine	0.030			<0.003	<0.01	<1
Monoidotyrosine	< 0.02			<0.002	<0.01	<1
Potassium iodide	< 0.0003					<0.05
Thyroglobulin (unhydrolyzed)	< 0.0003					<1

[a] Relative cross-reactivity is an arbitrary value if D,L-rT_3 or L-rT_3 were set at 100.
[b] D, L isomers.

Since the nature of serum protein binding of rT_3 was not known at the time, the approach adopted for rT_3 RIA consisted of the measurement of rT_3 in ethanol extracts of sera in a manner similar to that used by Patel et al. (1973 a) for T_3 RIA. Studies indicated that rT_3 is, indeed, a component of normal human serum and thyroglobulin, and the metabolism of T_4 is its most important source.

Several RIAs of rT_3 in serum have now been developed; many employ blocking agents, in a manner similar to those for RIA of T_3 and T_4, in order to displace rT_3 from binding proteins in serum and to inhibit the interference of serum proteins. The experiences with rT_3 RIA have been similar to those for T_3 RIA described previously. The mean normal serum rT_3 measured by different RIAs has varied substantially, ranging from 18 to 60 ng/dl. The differences in values may be attributed partially to the nature (D, L-rT_3 vs. L-rT_3) and purity of the rT_3 standards (Premchandra 1978). However, technical differences and difficulties are probably the main reason for the differences and should serve to remind us that the available rT_3 RIAs, while all reasonably precise, indicate a relative rather than absolute truth and that their major virtue is to be able to compare (apparently quite accurately) the relative changes in rT_3 in different circumstances.

The reagents and procedures of a convenient RIA of rT_3 in ethanol extracts of sera are outlined below; details have been published elsewhere (Chopra 1974).

1. Reverse T_3 Radioimmunoassay

a) Reagents

Anti-rT_3 antibody. Anti-rT_3 antibodies, produced as described above, may be tested for a dilution suitable for use in RIA and for specificity in the same manner as noted above for T_3 RIA. The specificity data on several published rT_3 RIAs are shown in Table 3.4. It is evident that anti-rT_3 antisera have the potential of remarkable specificity. Only 3,3′-T_2 shows a potentially worrisome cross-reaction (up to 10%) in rT_3 RIA, but its concentration in serum or thyroid is fortunately much too low compared with rT_3 to be a serious problem (Wu et al. 1976; Burman et al. 1977 a; Burger and Sakaloff 1977; Gavin et al. 1977).

Radioactive (^{125}I)-rT_3. This may be prepared in the laboratory by radioiodination of 3,3′-T_2 using chloramine T (Weeke and Orskov 1973; Burger and Ingbar 1974; Nakamura et al. 1977) or may be obtained from commercial sources (Abbott Laboratories, North Chicago, Ill.).

Reagent grade rT_3. This may be obtained from Henning, Berlin, West Germany.

b) Procedure

Add the various reagents to 10 × 75 mm glass disposable culture tubes in the following order: (1) 0.075 *M* barbital buffer (or phosphate buffered saline: 0.01 *M* phosphate, 0.14 *M* sodium chloride, pH 7.4) containing 1% normal rabbit serum and 0.01% sodium azide (assay buffer); (2) 300 µl of ethanol extract of a hormone-free serum (pooled serum of normal subjects, treated with activated charcoal) in tubes for standard curve, and an equal volume of an ethanol extract of test sera (prepared by mixing 1 ml 95% ethanol with 0.5 ml serum, followed by centrifugation at 1000 × *g* for 10 min; the supernatant is used directly in the assay); (3) unlabeled rT_3, 100 µl, containing 5 pg to 3 ng in tubes for standard curve; T_3 may be dissolved in 0.01 *M* NaOH and then diluted in assay buffer for use in RIA; (4) an appropriate dilution of anti-rT_3, 100 µl; (5) 100 µl of assay buffer containing approximately 10000 cpm of (^{125}I)-rT_3 (~10–30 pg rT_3).

The tubes are mixed and incubated at 4° C for 24 h. A sufficient amount of a previously titered second antibody, e. g., goat antirabbit γ-globulin, is then added to precipitate anti-rT_3-bound radioactive rT_3. Subsequent procedures for separation of bound from free radioactivity, correction for nonspecific binding of radioactivity, plotting of a standard curve, and using the standard curve to determine the results of rT_3 concentration in unknowns are the same as described for RIA of T_3.

B. Serum T_3 Concentration in Health and Disease

I. Age-Related Changes

Serum concentrations of T_3s (T_3 and rT_3) are influenced by their thyroidal secretion, by extrathyroidal metabolism of T_4 and T_3s, and by serum protein binding and the metabolic clearance rate of T_3s. These factors differ at various stages of life, hence the differences in serum levels of T_3s.

1. Fetal and Neonatal Life

Compared with the adult, serum T_3 concentration is typically reduced in the fetus and the newborn, whereas serum rT_3 concentration is increased (Chopra 1974; Chopra et al. 1975 a, b). Studies in the sheep suggest that low serum T_3 in the fetus results from a combination of at least two factors: (1) decreased extrathyroidal conversion of T_4 to T_3 and (2) increased metabolic clearance rate of T_3; the thyroidal secretion of T_3 seems well maintained in the fetus. High serum rT_3 concentration in the fetus also seems to result from at least two factors: (1) a reduction in the metabolic clearance rate of rT_3 and (2) an increase in the production rate of T_4; the conversion of T_4 to rT_3 in the fetus is well preserved and comparable to the adult (Fig. 4.2, Chopra et al. 1975 b; Wu et al. 1978 c).

The finding of low serum T_3 and high T_3 in the fetus compared with the adult has raised several interesting questions: (1) When does low T_3 and high rT_3 in the newborn become comparable to that of the normal adult? In other words, when does fetal metabolism of iodothyronines mature to normal adult levels? (2) How soon in fetal life are abnormal serum levels of iodothyronine manifested? (3) What are the factors responsible for a different metabolism of iodothyronines in the fetus compared with the adult? (4) Are there situations in the adult where iodothyronine metabolism reverts to that occurring normally in fetal life and, if so, what is their basis and/or function? Answers to these and related questions are not yet complete, but some interesting information has become available in recent years.

The following discussion pertains to the first three points cited above. The fourth point has been answered in the affirmative and will be discussed later in the section dealing with the effect of systemic illnesses, nutrition, and drugs on serum levels of T_3 and rT_3.

The answer to the first question, concerning the time when fetal metabolism of iodothyronines, is that low serum total T_3 matures to adult levels and the amount that is free in the fetus increases to values similar to or greater than those in the adult within a few hours after birth (Fig. 4.3, Abuid et al. 1974, Erenberg et al. 1974). The

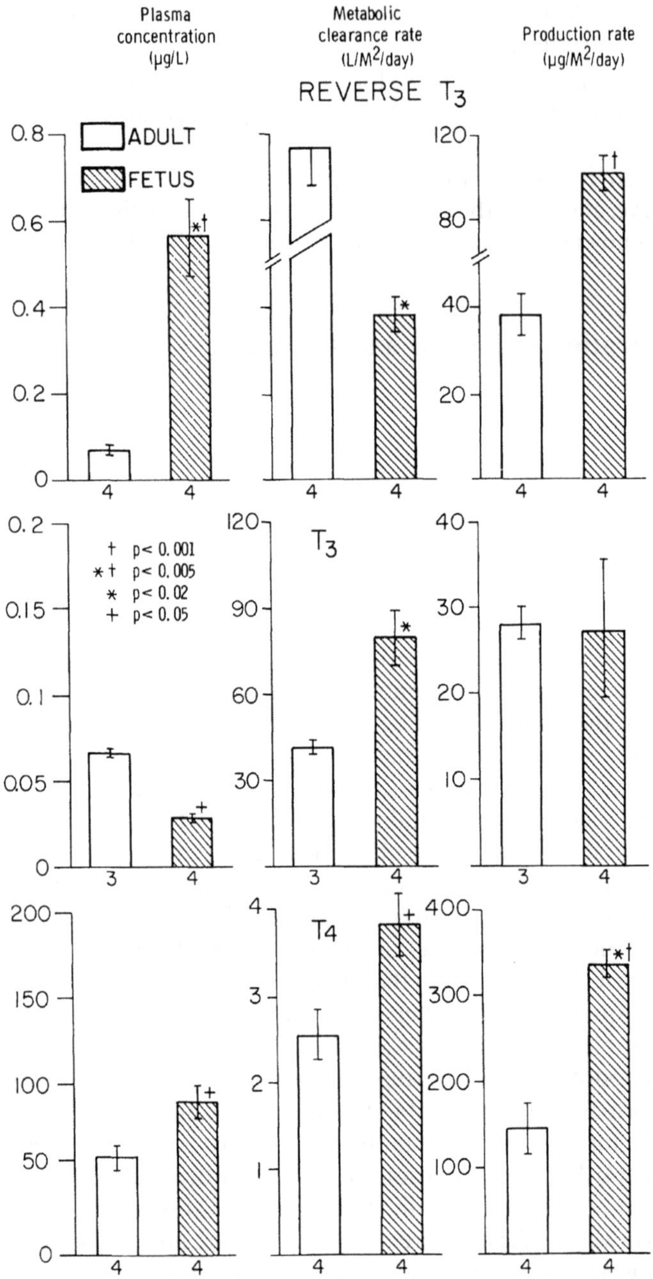

Fig. 4.2. Comparison of plasma concentration, MCR, and daily PR of T_3, T_3, and T_4 in fetal and adult sheep. Data from Chopra et al. 1975 b. (Chopra et al. 1978 c)

increase in the serum concentration of T_3 during the neonatal period is more pronounced than that in serum T_4. It results from at least two factors. Firstly, an abrupt marked increase in serum TSH from a cord serum value of about 9 μU/ml to about 80 μU/ml within 30 min of birth, and secondly a marked increase in the ability

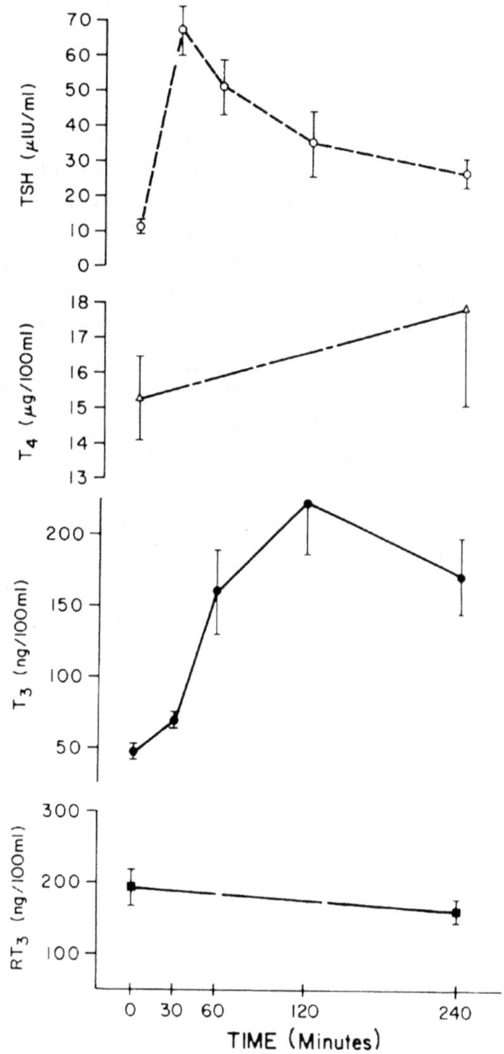

Fig. 4.3. Changes in serum thyrotropin (TSH) and iodothyronines (T_4, T_3, and rT_3) in neonatal period. Data from eight infants have been plotted as mean ± S.E.M. (Fisher et al. 1977)

of fetal tissues to convert T_4 to T_3 within a few hours of birth (Wu et al. 1978 c). The increase in serum TSH in the neonatal period appears related in part at least to the neonatal cooling that occurs after birth. The increase in serum T_3 concentration in the newborn seems to be linked, in addition to the TSH surge, to cord cutting, although the mechanism remains uncertain (Fisher and Odell 1969; Fisher et al. 1977). Recent studies show that tissue nonprotein sulfhydryl groups are vital to their ability to convert T_4 to T_3 and that there is an association of increased hepatic nonprotein sulfhydryl groups and increased T_4 to T_3 converting activity. In addition, it is possible that increased synthesis of $T_4 5'$-monodeiodinase is involved, to a degree, in increased conversion of T_4 to T_3 in neonatal tissues (Wu et al. 1978 c; Segall-Blank 1978; Chopra 1978 b).

Contrary to T_3, high serum rT_3 concentration in the newborn remains high compared with adult values for several days. Serum rT_3 does not increase appreciably during the period of the TSH surge, probably because thyroidal secretion normally contributes minimally to circulating rT_3. Serum rT_3 declines gradually to or toward normal adult levels by the 2nd week of life in man (Fig. 4.4).

Just as in man, serum rT_3 is elevated in the fetal rat compared with the adult rat, and it declines progressively to reach low adult levels in the first few days ($\sim$7 days) of postnatal life (Harris et al. 1978). However, normalization of high serum rT_3 in sheep may be delayed until 4–6 weeks of postnatal life (Chopra et al. 1975 b). Studies in sheep suggest that the process of normalization of high serum rT_3 (and low T_3) in the fetus actually begins a few (3–6) days prior to spontaneous parturition and that it is associated with an increase in plasma cortisol (Klein et al. 1978). Cortisol infusion in the sheep fetus has been shown to be associated with an increase in T_4 to T_3 converting activity in the liver (Wu et al. 1978 c). This effect of glucocorticoids in the sheep fetus is different from that in the adult, in whom glucocorticoid administration is associated with a reduction in serum T_3 and an increase in serum rT_3, apparently resulting from a reduction in iodothyronine 5′-monodeiodinating activities (Duick et al. 1974; Chopra et al. 1975 c).

The question concerning at what time during fetal life the characteristic serum levels of T_3s first become evident has not yet been answered adequately. T_3 is detectable in low levels (20 ng/dl) in the serum of a human fetus at about 25 weeks of gestation; and its concentration increases to about 50 ng/dl at 40 weeks gestation (normal range, 50–210 ng/dl in nonpregnant adults and 160 to 300 ng/dl in pregnant

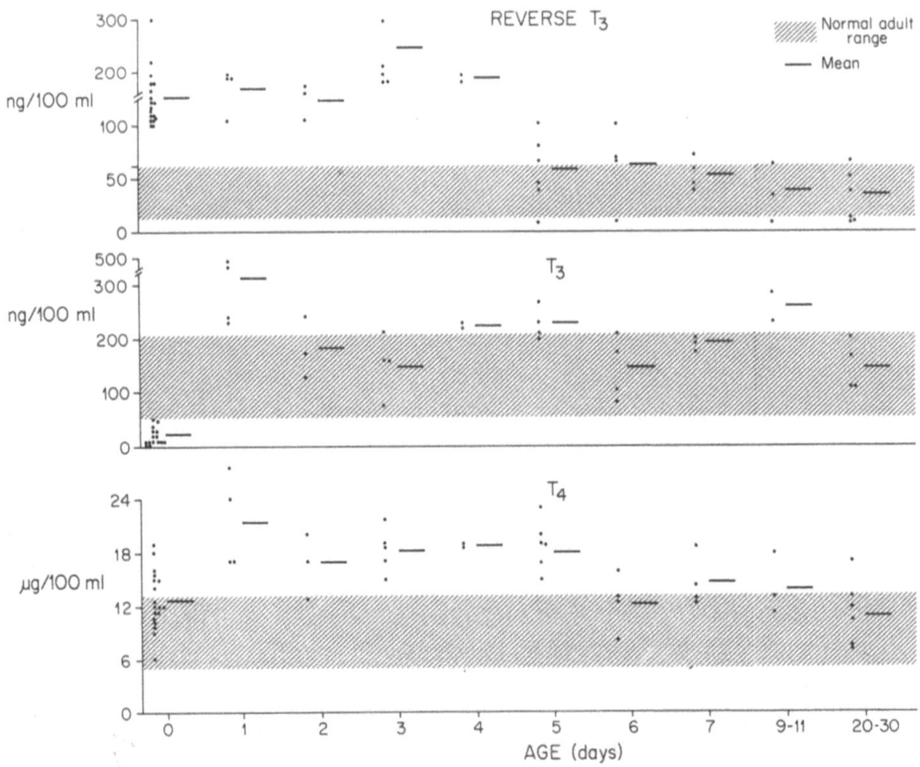

Fig. 4.4. Serum concentration of thyroid hormones from birth to 30 days of life. Data from Chopra et al. 1975 a. (Chopra 1978 a)

women). Similar data are not available on serum rT_3 concentration during intrauterine life. However, rT_3 is easily detectable in a very high concentration in amniotic fluid at 15–19 weeks gestation. In a recent study, amniotic fluid rT_3 concentration averaged 330 ng/dl at 15–19 weeks gestation and declined to a mean value of 93 ng/dl at 36–42 weeks gestation (Fig. 4.5). These values compare with those in maternal sera of 58 ng/dl at 15–16 weeks pregnancy and 59 ng/dl at 35–42 weeks pregnancy (Chopra and Crandall 1975). These data suggested that rT_3 should be detectable and may possibly be elevated in the circulation of a human fetus within a few weeks of onset of thyroidal function, and the detectability of T_4 has been documented at 11 weeks gestation (Greenberg et al. 1970). The serum concentration of T_3s has been documented more accurately in the sheep fetus. As in man, serum T_3 concentration in this species is low throughout gestation, whereas serum rT_3 is elevated as early as 90 days gestation (normal gestation period in sheep is about 145 days) (Fisher et al. 1977).

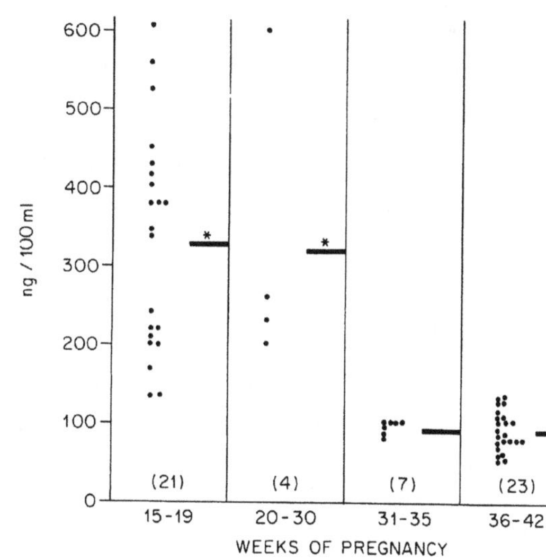

Fig. 4.5. Reverse T_3 concentration amniotic fluid at varius stages of pregnancy. (Reprinted with permission from Chopra and Crandall 1975)

2. Childhood (1–15 Years of Age)

Recent studies indicate that serum T_3 (and T_4) concentrations decrease progressively with age between 1 and 15 years (Fisher et al. 1978). A similar gradual decline in serum-T_3 with age has also been documented in some (Rubenstein et al. 1973), but not in other, previous studies (Av Ruskin et al. 1973). However, the number of children (~50) in the study of Av Ruskin et al. was much smaller than that (195) in the study of Fisher et al. (1978).

The fall in serum T_3 (and T_4) between 1 and 15 years of age seems related mainly to the associated fall in the serum concentration of TBG during this time, when mean serum TBG, T_3, and T_4 concentrations decrease about 30%, 29%, and 31%, respectively (Fisher et al. 1978). Curiously, however, free T_3 and free T_4 index values also decreased with age in the study of Fisher et al. (1978). The fall in the free T_4 index with age was not observed in another study (Shenkman and Hollander 1975).

However, the observation of a progressive decrease in T_4 turnover with age during adolescence and childhood (Fisher and Dussault 1974) supports the occurrence of a fall in free T_4 concentration at this age. Similar data are not yet available on T_3 turnover.

Unlike the fall in serum T_3 concentration, a slight increase in serum rT_3 concentration has been observed in children between 1 and 15 years of age. No data are yet available on turnover rates of rT_3 during this time. Therefore, it is not known whether the observed modest increase in serum rT_3 during these years is due to increased production, decreased metabolic clearance of rT_3, or a combination of both factors (Fisher et al. 1978).

3. Adult Life

As in children between 1 and 15 years of age, a decrease in serum T_3 (and/or T_4) concentration and an increase in serum rT_3 concentration with aging has been documented in several studies of adult subjects (Brunell and Bohuon 1972; Rubenstein et al. 1973; Mlholm et al. 1975; Hesch et al. 1976; Westgren et al. 1976; Nicod et al. 1976; Chopra and Solomon 1976). However, in a more recent and careful study, it was suggested that advancement in age, per se, is not accompanied by changes in serum concentration of total or free T_3 (and T_4) and total rT_3, and that the previously reported effects of age on serum T_3, rT_3, or T_4 may have been influenced by coexisting, and possibly unidentified, systemic illness or by ingestion of some drugs (Olsen et al. 1978). The data on the effects of systemic illnesses and/or drugs on serum iodothyronines are reviewed below.

II. Effect of Sex

Serum T_3 (or T_4) or rT_3 concentrations do not differ appreciably in men and women except during pregnancy, at which time the increase in serum TBG concentration is associated with an increase in the serum concentration of both T_3s and of T_4 (Chopra and Solomon 1976; Chopra 1974; Olsen et al. 1978). Similarly, serum T_3 and rT_3 (and T_4) concentrations are low when the serum concentration of TBG is low, as in euthyroid patients with malnutrition, during androgen adminsitration, or when there is genetic defect in the synthesis of TBG.

III. Effect of Thyroid Disease

Typically, serum concentrations of T_3, rT_3, and T_4 are increased in hyperthyroidism. However, the levels overlap and there are normal values in each case. Normal concentrations are minimal for serum T_3 values in hyperthyroidism. The overlap with normal values is quite marked for both T_3 and rT_3 in hypothyroidism; serum T_4 is more discriminating in this case.

1. Hyperthyroidism

The mean T_3 concentration is increased (about four-to six fold) in the hyperthyroidism of Graves' disease to a much greater degree than is serum T_4 (two- to fourfold); the increase in mean serum rT_3 concentration is usually similar to that in serum T_4 (Figs. 4.6, 4.7, 4.8). The reason for an unusual increase in the serum T_3

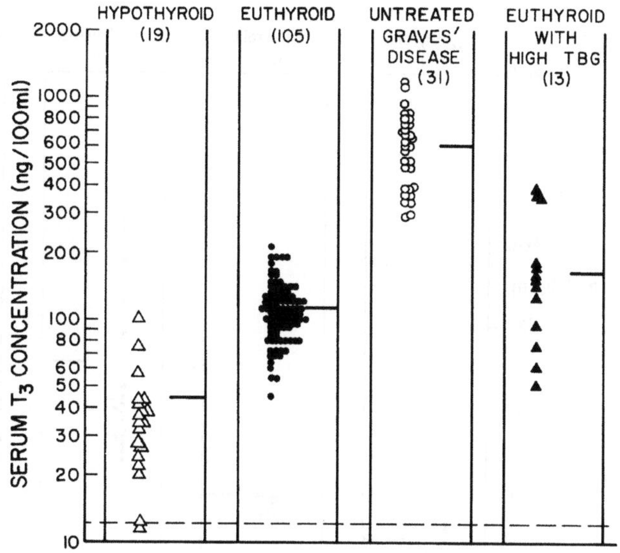

Fig. 4.6. Serum T_3 concentration, as measured by RIA, in normal subjects and patients with hypothyroidism and hyperthyroidism. (Reprinted with permission from Chopra and Solomon 1976) [Pharmacol Ther [B] I. Chopra IJ, Solomon DH. Thyroid function tests and their alterations by drugs] Copyright 1976, Pergamon Press, Ltd.

concentration of hyperthyroidism appears related to a higher concentration of T_3, relative to that of T_4, in the thyroid gland. Thus, the molar ration of T_4 and T_3 (T_4/T_3) in thyroglobulin was observed to be (mean $\pm$ S. D.) 9.0 ± 2.0 in patients with treated Graves' disease, 3.4 ± 1.0 in patients treated with antithyroid drugs, and 15 ± 2.0 in normal subjects. The concentration of T_3 in the thyroglobulin of patients

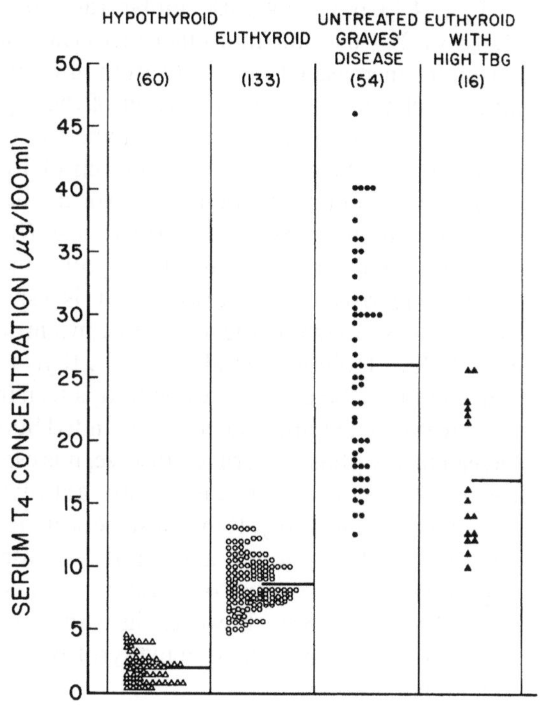

Fig. 4.7. Serum T_4 concentration measured by RIA in euthyroid subjects and patients with hypothyroidism and hyperthyroidism. Reprinted with permission from [Pharmacol Ther [B] I. Chopra IJ, Solomon DH. Thyroid function tests and their alterations by drugs] Copyright 1976, Pergamon Press, Ltd.

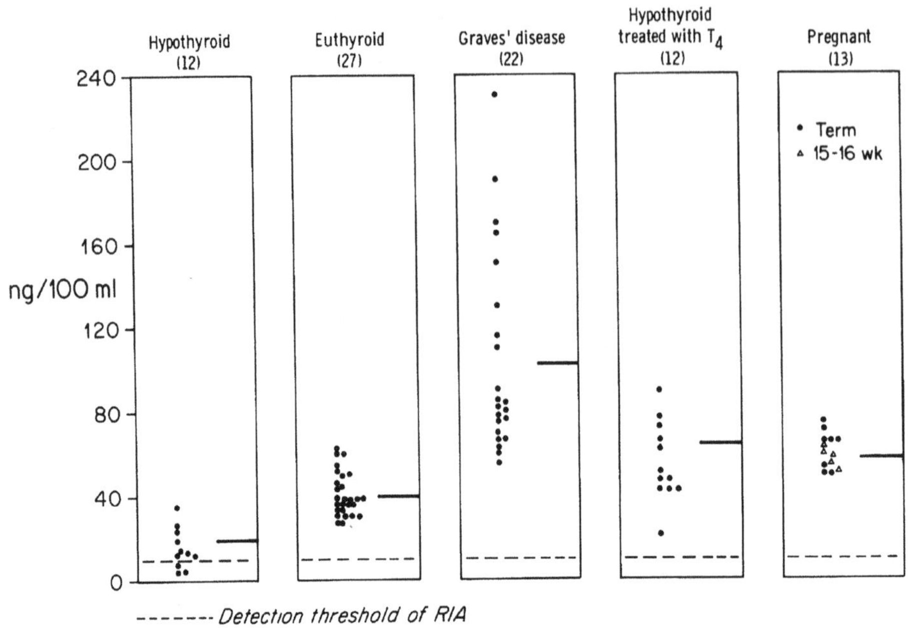

Fig. 4.8. Serum concentration of T_3 as measured by RIA in health and thyroid disease. Date from Chopra (1974), Chopra and Crandall (1975), Chopra et al. (1978 c). Reprinted by permission. Figure taken from Chopra et al. 1978 c

with untreated Graves' disease was above normal even when the concentration of T_4 (3.4 ± 0.6 vs. 3.4 ± 0.8, molar ratio of T_4 and thyroglobulin) and iodine (29 ± 5 vs. 29 ± 6 atoms/molecule) were clearly normal (Izumi and Larsen 1977); the reason for increased T_3 concentration in Graves' thyroglobulin is not clear, but it may be related to hyperstimulation of the thyroid.

The serum concentration of T_3 in hyperthyroidism does not clearly correlate with the severity of the disorder. Serum levels of T_3 (or T_4, measured as protein-bound iodine) in patients with thyroid storm do not differ significantly from those in patients with uncomplicated thyrotoxicosis (Brooks et al. 1975). The measurement of serum T_3 concentration in hyperthyroidism may be the single most sensitive test in the diagnosis of this disorder. It is especially useful in patients with T_3-thyrotoxicosis in whom the serum T_4 concentration is within normal limits (Sterling et al. 1970 a; Hollander et al. 1972). T_3-thyrotoxicosis is more common in regions where iodine deficiency is prevalent. It is seen in about 5% of hyperthyroid patients in iodine sufficient areas such as the United States. Although T_3 thyrotoxicosis may be seen in any phase of Graves' disease, it is especially common during or following treatment of hyperthyroidism with antithyroid drugs, radioactive iodine, or subtotal thyroidectomy. It may also be seen in patients with solitary toxic adenoma and multinodular goiter and in those cases of thyrotoxicosis factitia where hyperthyroidism is a result of ingestion of T_3. Serum T_4 concentration is subnormal in the latter instances, however, instead of normal, as seen in other cases of T_3 thyrotoxicosis, or high, as seen in thyrotoxicosis factitia due to thyroid (USP) or T_4 ingestion.

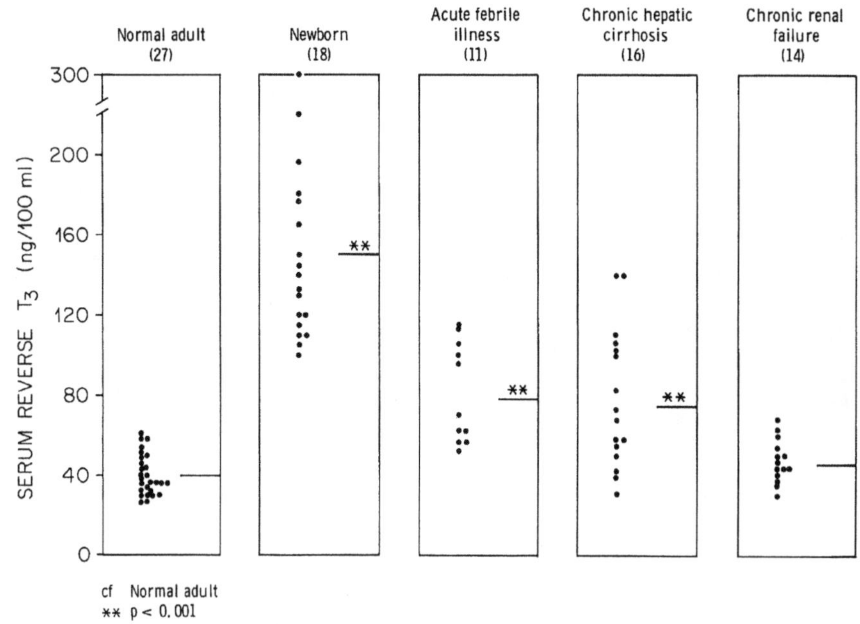

Fig. 4.9. Serum concentration of rT_3 in newborn cord blood and adult patients with various systemic illnesses. Significance compared with normal adult: $^{**}P < 0.001$. Data from Chopra et al. 1975 d. (Chopra et al. 1978 c)

The diagnostic accuracy of serum T_3 values is limited in a number of clinical situations including systemic illnesses and during administration of some drugs that are associated with a reduction in extrathyroidal conversion of T_4 to T_3. These situations are discussed in a later section of this volume.

Although, like serum T_3, the serum concentration of rT_3 is typically considerably elevated in hyperthyroidism, its measurement is neither necessary nor appropriate in the routine diagnosis of hyperthyroidism. High serum rT_3 concentration can be seen in euthyroid subjects with a wide variety of nonthyroidal systemic illnesses and during the administration of several drugs (Fig. 4.9). On the other hand, serum rT_3 concentration may be normal in up to 18% of hyperthyroid patients (Kaplan et al. 1977). The measurement of rT_3, however, provides insights into the situation when serum T_3 is normal and serum T_4 is high in hyperthyroid patients in whom extrathyroidal metabolism of T_4 to T_3 is reduced because of associated nonthyroid illnesses or drug ingestion. Even in these circumstances, however, laboratory tests, such as the thyrotropin releasing hormone stimulation test (TRH test) (Hershman and Pittman 1970) and/or the thyroid hormone suppression test (Werner and Spooner 1955; Wallack et al. 1970), provide better diagnostic information than the measurement of serum rT_3 concentration.

2. Hypothyroidism

Serum T_3 and rT_3 concentrations may be within the normal range in up to 20% and 40% of hypothyroid patients respectively; they are subnormal in the remaining cases (Fig. 4.10; Chopra et al. 1972 a, 1973 a; Larsen 1972; Kaplan et al. 1977). The

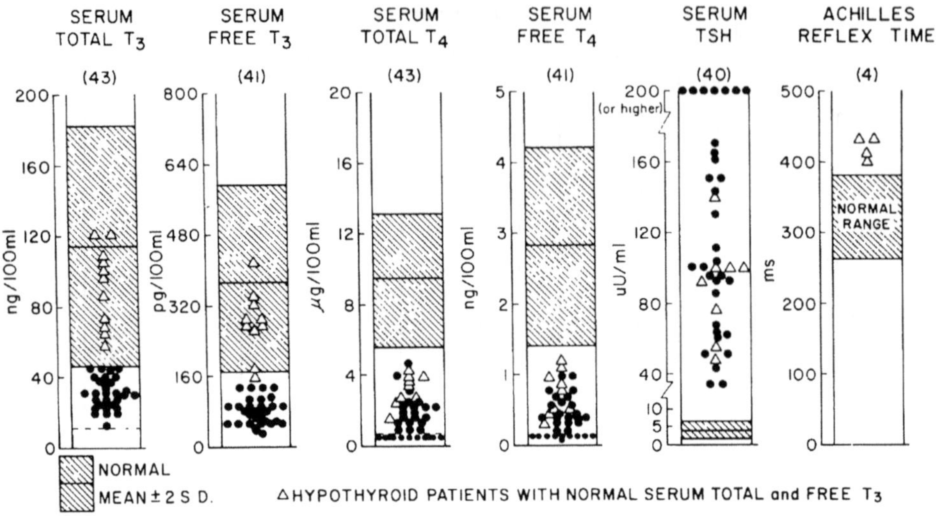

Fig. 4.10. Thyroid function tests in hypothyroidism. Data from Chopra et al. (1973 a)

normal concentration of T_3s in several cases with hypothyroidism may be related to hyperstimulation of a thyroidal remnant by elevated TSH and reduced iodination of thyroglobulin as well as to a reduction in metabolic clearance of T_3s. In any case, it is clear that measurement of neither T_3 nor rT_3 is very helpful in the routine diagnosis of hypothyroidism. The measurement of the serum concentration of T_4, its interpretation in the light of abnormalities in serum TBG concentration, if any, and serum TSH concentration measurement are appropriate ways to establish the diagnosis of hypothyroidism.

3. Chronic Thyroiditis

The serum concentrations of T_3, T_4, and rT_3 are usually normal in euthyroid individuals and subnormal in hypothyroid patients with chronic thyroiditis. In some cases, however, serum T_4 is borderline normal or low in clinically euthyroid patients, while serum T_3 is clearly normal or even slightly elevated; serum rT_3 levels usually follow the direction of serum T_4 levels. Serum TSH is elevated in such cases and is apparently responsible for sustaining euthyroidism by maintaining serum T_3 at high normal or high levels. There are other euthyroid patients with chronic thyroiditis in whom serum TSH is elevated even at a time when serum T_4 and T_3 levels are within normal limits. The mechanism of this combination of laboratory findings is not entirely clear. It is possible that elevated TSH is required to drive the diseased thyroid sufficiently to secrete normal levels of thyroid hormones, or that serum T_4 and T_3 concentrations, although within the normal range, are less than those present before the onset of thyroiditis. Finally, the possibility cannot be excluded that there is an abnormality in the pituitary–thyroid axis in chronic thyroiditis.

4. Endemic Goiter

Serum T_3 levels in inhabitants of endemic goiter regions where iodine deficiency is prevalent are typically normal or moderately elevated at a time when serum T_4 is low normal or low (De Lange et al. 1972; Patel et al. 1973 b; Pharoah et al. 1973; Kochupillai et al. 1973; Chopra et al. 1975 e). Normal serum T_3 levels thus provide an explanation for the apparent paradox of clinical euthyroidism despite subnormal T_4. Serum TSH is elevated in endemic goiter patients with low T_4. Interestingly, it correlates negatively better with serum T_4 levels than with serum T_3 levels (Figs. 4.11 and 4.12, Chopra et al. 1975 e). This finding suggested that T_4 may serve TSH-suppressive effects without prior conversion to T_3. This inference is presently not as apparent as it was in 1975. Silva et al. (1978) have recently demonstrated that T_4 can be converted in the rat pituitary to T_3 and that this local contribution of T_4 monodeiodination to T_3 may be very important to the pituitary nuclear content of T_3 and control of TSH secretion. One wonders, however, why clearly normal or even high serum T_3 levels in iodine deficiency states do not fill in, at equilibrium, the nuclear T_3 binding sites normally intended for occupation by T_3 derived from T_4 monodeiodination. In any case, until further information is available, one may consider that serum TSH is elevated in inhabitants of endemic goiter regions because T_4 is low and because the reduction in availability of T_4 as a substrate for conversion to T_3 results in a reduction in intrapituitary T_3 and T_3 in the pituitary nuclei.

Serum rT_3 levels have not been studied as well as serum T_3 in persons with endemic goiter. We have observed significantly low mean values in inhabitants of

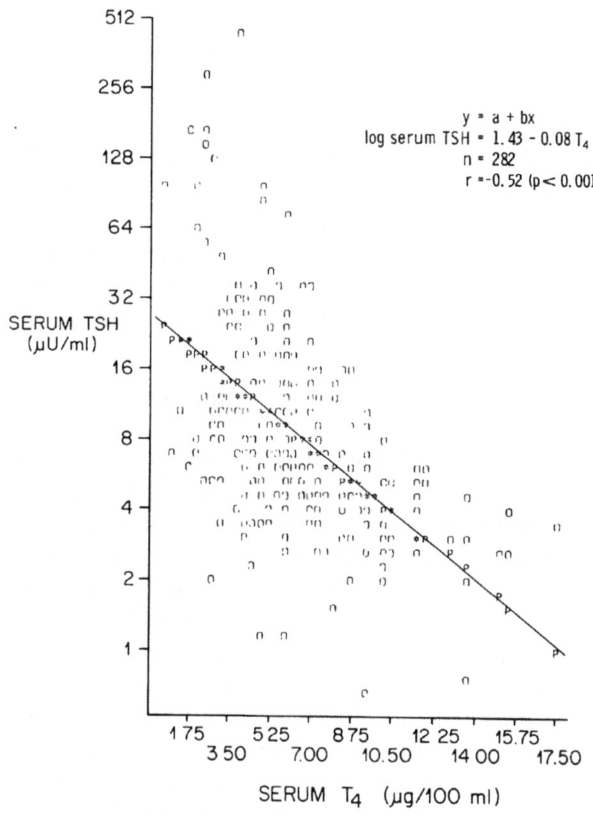

Fig. 4.11. Relationship between serum T_4 and TSH concentrations in inhabitants of an endemic goiter region of New Guinea. (Chopra et al. 1975 e)

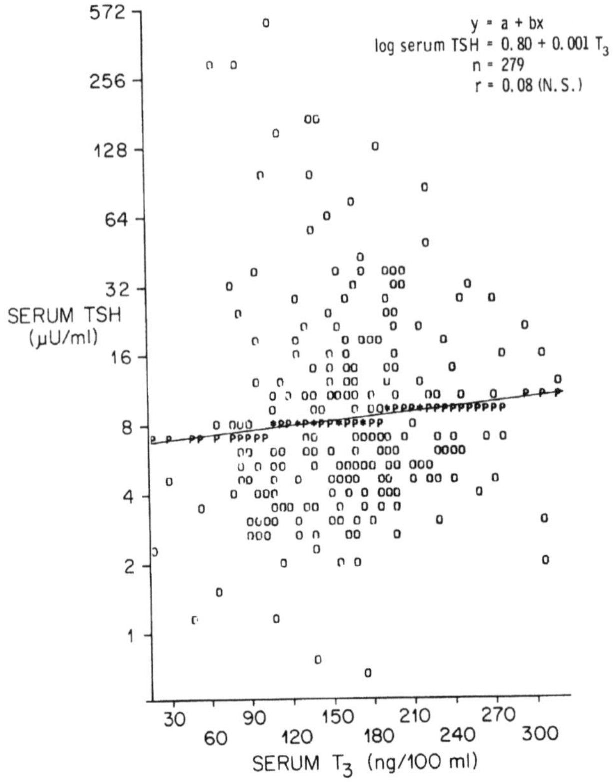

Fig. 4.12. Relationship between serum T_3 and TSH concentrations in inhabitants of an endemic goiter region of New Guinea. (Chopra et al. 1975 e)

the Nomane region of New Guinea in whom the mean serum T_4 levels was diminished, while mean serum T_3 and TSH levels were high (Chopra et al. 1975 e). Serum rT_3 tended to follow, in general, the direction of serum T_4, and there was no significant difference in the mean values of goitrous and nongoitrous subjects. In pregnant subjects from endemic goiter regions, serum rT_3 is high, as are serum T_3 and T_4 concentrations (Medeiros-Neto et al. 1978).

IV. Effect of Nonthyroidal Illnesses

A wide variety of nonthyroidal systemic illnesses and caloric-deprivation states are associated with an appreciable, and often dramatic, change in the serum concentration of iodothyronines (Table 4.4). Serum T_3 concentration is characteristically reduced in systemic illnesses while serum rT_3 concentration is characteristically increased (Figs. 4.9 and 4.13). Serum T_4 can be normal, high or low; low values are usually seen in critically ill patients. These changes in the serum concentration of iodothyronines occur beyond those explained by changes in serum concentrations of iodothyronine-binding proteins in systemic illnesses. Serum concentrations of free T_3 and rT_3 are also changed in the same direction as are total T_3 and rT_3. Serum free T_4 concentration, as measured by equilibrium dialysis, is normal or high in the majority of the patients; it can also be subnormal in a few very seriously ill patients (Figs. 4.13 and 4.14, Chopra et al. 1974, 1979 a).

Table 4.4. Some clinical situations with low-T_3 syndrome, i.e., clinical euthyroidism with low serum total and/or free T_3, and normal total T_4 and/or normal or high serum free T_4 and high total and/or free rT_3

Clinical situation	References
Calorie deprivation states	
Complete fasting	Portnay et al. 1974; Vagenakis et al. 1975; Spaulding et al. 1976; Carlson et al. 1977; Eisenstein et al. 1978; Suda et al. 1978 a, b
Protein–calorie malnutrition	Rastogi et al. 1974; Chopra and Smith 1975
Anorexia nervosa	Miyai et al. 1975; Moshang et al. 1975; Croxson and Ibberston 1977
Systemic illnesses	
Febrile states	Chopra et al. 1975c; Wartofsky et al. 1977
Diabetes mellitus	Naeije et al. 1976; Piroska and Foldes 1976; Suda et al. 1977
Hepatic cirrhosis	Chopra et al. 1974; 1975c; Nomura et al. 1975
Renal failure	Fang et al. 1974; Chopra et al. 1975c
Myocardial infarction	Kaplan et al. 1977; Smith et al. 1978
Miscellaneous illnesses	Reichlin et al. 1973; Carter et al. 1974; Chopra et al. 1975d; Bermudez et al. 1975; McLarty et al. 1975; Burger et al. 1976b; Burrows et al. 1977
Toxemia of pregnancy	Osathanondh et al. 1976
Burns	Becker et al. 1976
Surgical operations	Burr et al. 1975; Brandt et al. 1976
Drugs	
Dexamethasone	Duick et al. 1974; Chopra et al. 1975a; Burr et al. 1976; DeGroot and Haye 1976; Westgren et al. 1977b
Radiocontrast agents for cholecytography – Telepaque, Oragrafin	Burgi et al. 1976; Wu et al. 1978a, b
Antianginal agent, Amiodarone	Burger et al. 1976a
Propylthiouracil	Saberi et al. 1975; Geffner et al. 1975; Westgren et al. 1977a; Kaplan et al. 1977; Laurberg and Weeke 1978
Propranolol	Wiersinga and Touber 1977; Verhoeven et al. 1977

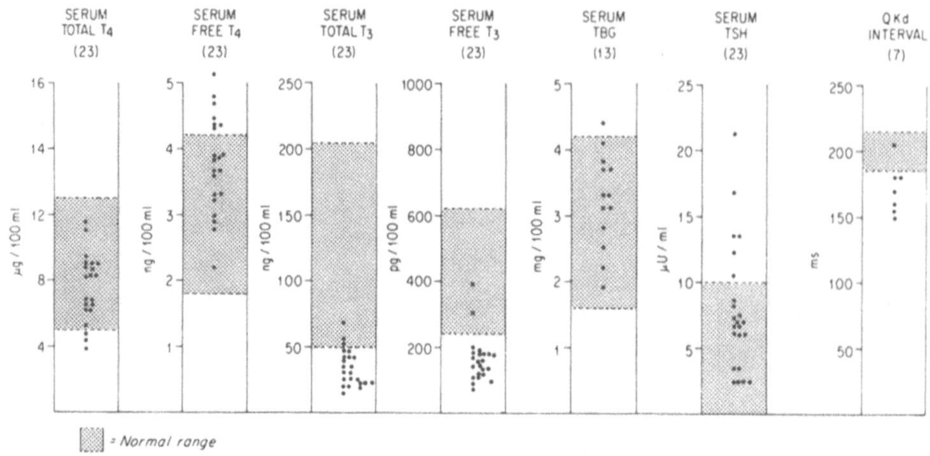

Fig. 4.13. Serum concentration of thyroid hormones and TSH and QKd intervals in patients with hepatic cirrhosis. QKd interval represents the interval between beginning of QRS complex in electrocardiogram (EKG) and the appearance of the first Korotkoff sound over the brachial artery when EKG and blood pressure are recorded simultaneously. Characteristically, QKd interval decreases in hyperthyroidism and increases in hypothyroidism. Stippled areas represent the normal response range. Data from Chopra et al. (1974). (Chopra et al. 1978c)

The term "low-T_3 syndrome" has been used to describe the above-mentioned biochemical findings in clinically euthyroid patients with nonthyroidal illnesses. The name, in part, is derived from the initial studies of Sullivan et al. (1973), who observed that T_3 levels are low in the tissues as well as in the sera of clinically euthyroid patients dying from a variety of serious systemic illnesses. More recent studies indicate that serum T_3 concentration and T_3 production rate are subnormal in low-T_3 syndrome while serum T_4 concentration is high, normal, or low; free T_4 concentration is normal or high (and rarely low); and T_4 production is normal or low (Chopra et al. 1975d; Chopra 1976a; Suda et al. 1977, 1978a, b). The serum TSH level is typically in the normal range and sometimes slightly elevated in this syndrome. Serum TSH response to TRH is also usually normal; responses that are slightly above or below normal have been reported in a few cases, however (Chopra et al. 1974; Bermudez et al. 1975; Vinik et al. 1975; Green et al. 1977). Normal serum TSH levels and the TSH response to TRH in the majority of patients are consistent with the clinical impression of euthyroidism.

Identification of the low-T_3 syndrome has raised many interesting and important clinical, as well as physiologic, questions. These include the following: (1) Are the patients with low-T_3 syndrome euthyroid or hypothyroid? (2) If they are euthyroid, how is this normal state maintained? (3) Is euthyroidism maintained by an increase in free T_4 concentration, observed in many cases, compensating for the reduced free T_3 concentration, or is there an increase in the sensitivity of thyroid hormone responsive tissues in nonthyroid illness? (4) Since serum concentrations of both T_3 and T_4 are low in some patients with nonthyroid illnesses, what are the appropriate clinical tests for assessment of thyroid function in the presence of nonthyroid illnesses? (5) What are the physiologic changes responsible for alterations in characteristic serum concentrations of T_3 and rT_3 (i.e., low-T_3 and high-rT_3) in

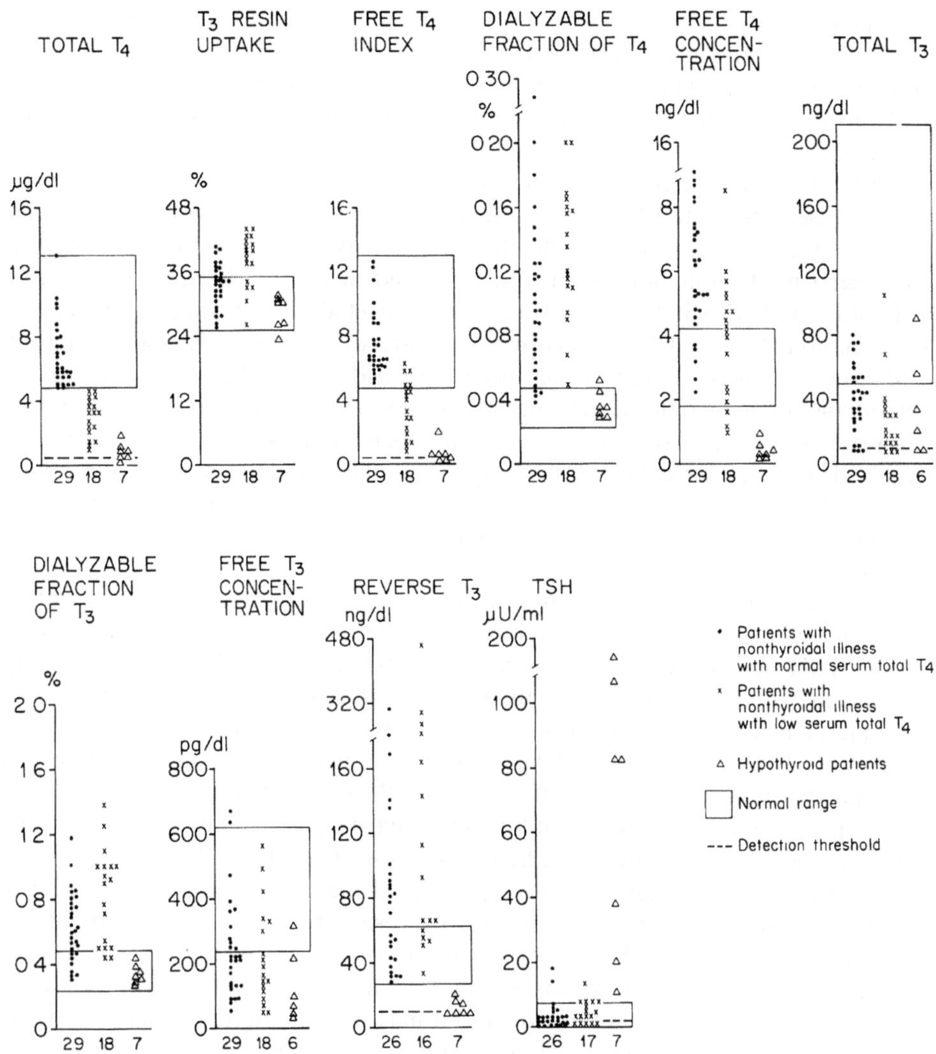

Fig. 4.14. Comparison of thyroid function test data in patients with nonthyroid illness with normal T_4, with low T_4, and in hypothyroid patients. (Chopra et al. 1979 a)

nonthyroid illness? (6) Do these physiologic alterations in iodothyronine metabolism (and resulting changes in iodothyronine levels in circulation) occur because they serve a homeostatic function or do they simply reflect a metabolic alterations because the tissues concerned with the metabolism are no longer healthy? (7) What is the signal which turns on the characteristic alterations in iodothyronine metabolism in nonthyroid illness? These are just a few examples of the varied questions that may be raised. Answers to most of these and similar questions are presently either incomplete or unavailable. We do not even know at this time whether the physiologic basis for all causes of the low-T_3 syndrome is the same or whether many different mechanisms are involved. In any case, a brief discussion of answers to the above-mentioned questions follows.

It has generally been assumed that the metabolic basis for the low-T_3 syndrome is an alteration in the metabolism of T_4, whereby its monodeiodination in the outer ring to T_3 is reduced while that in the inner ring to rT_3 remains normal. The reduced daily production rate of T_3 has been confirmed in some conditions with the low-T_3 syndrome, e. g., in fetal life and in adults undergoing complete fasting or those suffering from hepatic cirrhosis (Chopra et al. 1975 b; Chopra 1976 a; Suda et al. 1978 a; Eisenstein et al. 1978), and it appears likely in other conditions not yet fully studied. High serum rT_3 is explained by increased availability of the substrate, T_4, for inner ring deiodination (to rT_3) and reduced metabolic clearance rate of rT_3 (Chopra et al. 1975 a, b; Chopra 1976 a; Eisenstein et al. 1978; Suda et al. 1978). The combination of reduced T_4 to T_3 conversion and reduced metabolism of rT_3 in most situations with low-T_3 syndrome has been explained by considering that the same 5′ (outer ring) monodeiodinase acts on both T_4 and rT_3 (Kaplan and Utiger 1978 a). However, the issue of one versus two 5′-monodeiodinases has not yet been fully resolved; it is discussed further in Chap. 8. Similarly, the mechanism of reduced tissue activity of T_4 5′-monodeiodinase has been studied in only a few examples of low-T_3 syndrome, e. g., fetus and fasting adult. These studies are reviewed in Chap. 8.

The question of whether patients with the low-T_3 syndrome are euthyroid or hypothyroid has also been answered only in a limited fashion as yet. The data on serum TSH and serum TSH response (see above) are variable but are mostly consistent with euthyroid status in patients with low-T_3 syndrome. Similarly, peripheral metabolic indices, e. g., Achilles reflex time and QKd interval, i. e., time elapsed between the onset of the QRS complex in the electrocardiogram (ECG) and the appearence of a Korotkoff sound over the brachial artery, when ECG and blood pressure are recorded simultaneously, have suggested euthyroidism in the low-T_3 syndrome associated with hepatic cirrhosis (Fig. 4.13, Chopra et al. 1974). However, findings suggesting reduced peripheral effects of thyroid hormones have been recorded in patients with anorexia nervosa (Croxson and Ibbertson 1977). Oxygen consumption (BMR) has not been studied extensively in the low-T_3 syndrome, apparently because this parameter is influenced considerably by several factors unrelated to thyroid function and it may be even more unreliable than the parameters already mentioned. Thus, although the evidence is not definite, studies do suggest that it is possible to sustain euthyroidism even when serum T_3 is low. It is possible that the euthyroidism is maintained by high normal or high free T_4 concentration. There is little evidence to suggest increased sensitivity of tissues to thyroid hormones in low-T_3 syndrome. Studies using the fragments of the anterior pituitary gland of the fasting rat have not suggested any appreciable increase in the sensitivity of thyrotrope to thyroid hormone effects in fasting (Chopra et al. 1978 b).

Thyroid function studies in patients with systemic illnesses have revealed some clinically important diagnostic problems. In some cases, serum T_4 concentration is elevated and raises the question of hyperthyroidism even though serum in T_3 is low-normal or low and hypermetabolism and goiter are not present. The recovery from the underlying illness is associated with normalization of high serum T_4 (as well as low serum T_3) levels (Birkhauser et al. 1977; Gavin and Rosenthal 1977). Thyroid hormone suppression and/or TRH stimulation tests may be necessary to differentiate hyperthyroidism clearly from systemic illness. Conversely, although free T_4 concentration is generally normal or high, there are several clinically euthyroid patients with systemic illness in whom serum T_4 is low, thereby raising a question of hypothyroidism. Furthermore, just as total T_4, the free T_4 index is low (Fig. 4.14) and does not alleviate the diagnostic dilemma of hypothyroidism. Serum TSH is usually normal, providing an argument against the diagnosis of primary hypothyroidism, but the possibility of secondary hypothyroidism cannot be excluded. The serum of rT_3 is usually high-normal or clearly high in systemic illness and low-normal or clearly low in hypothyroidism. The measurement of rT_3 and/or free T_4 concentration may thus be useful in the diagnosis of hypothyroidism (Chopra et al. 1979 a).

It is not clear why in systemic illnesses values of "free T_4" assessed by the free T_4 index (from the T_3 resin uptake test) are lower than those assessed by the free T_4 concentration (from the dialyzable fraction of T_4 measured by equilibrium dialysis). A recent study suggests that there is an inhibitor of thyroid hormone-binding to serum proteins in the circulation of some patients with nonthyroid illnesses (Chopra et al. 1979 b). It is possible that the inhibitor functions well under the conditions of equilibrium dialysis but not under those of T_3 resin uptake. More study is needed.

The physiologic purpose to a reduction of T_3 in the low-T_3 syndrome is not clear. It is interesting to note, however, that tissue catabolism is increased in most cases of low-T_3 syndrome where the conversion of T_4 to T_3 is reduced. This is not true of the fetus but in this case tissue catabolism is clearly undesirable and conservation of nutrients is necessary for the sake of optimal growth and development. Occurrence of the low-T_3 syndrome during the administration of some drugs, e.g., X-ray contrast agents, propylthiouracil, and possibly Amiodarone (2-n-Butyl-3-(4′-diethylaminoethoxy-3′,5′-diiodobenzoyl)-benzofurane, Cordarone, Labaz Inc., Brussels, Belgium) and propranolol may be a result of the interaction between the drug and the T_4 5′-monodeiodinase enzyme (see Chap. 8).

Hypothyroidism leads to growth retardation and hyperthyroidism is associated with a negative nitrogen balance. It has been demonstrated that T_4, T_3, rT_3, and 3,3′-T_2 are all able to stimulate amino acid uptake by thymocytes in vitro (Goldfine et al. 1976) and therefore they may all possess anabolic functions. A study was conducted in the rat to determine whether T_4, T_3, and rT_3, or only some of the iodothyronines, possess catabolic properties evidenced by their ability to cause a negative nitrogen balance (Chopra et al. 1978 c). The results suggested that T_4 and rT_3 have little or no catabolic effect and that the catabolic effect of T_4 may result largely from its conversion to T_3 in extrathyroidal tissues (Fig. 4.15). These data favor the thesis that there is a homeostatic "wisdom" in the natural arrangement, whereby conversion of T_4 to T_3 is inhibited when tissue catabolism is enhanced. The change in the metabolism thus appears to support the survival of the organism. Preliminary clinical studies in fasting human subjects also support this analysis. Thus, normalization of low serum T_3 levels in fasting human subjects by exogenous T_3 administration was associated with an increase in muscle catabolism and release of muscle glutamine and 3-methylhistidine as well as an increase in urinary urea and ammonia nitrogen excretion; serum TSH response to TRH was also blunted and was consistent with hyperthyroidism (Vignati et al. 1978; Gardner et al. 1979). Overall, the available evidence in the low-T_3 syndrome favors a protein-sparing and homeostatic purpose for the reduction in serum T_3 rather than that it is an unrelated side effect of the illness resulting from the disease-induced limitation in the ability of the tissues to convert T_4 to T_3.

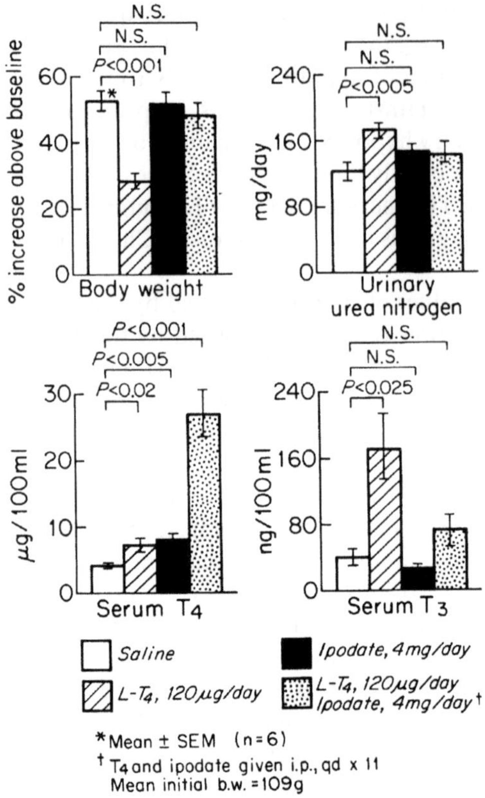

Fig. 4.15. Evidence suggesting a lack of catabolic effect of T_4 when its conversion to T_3 is inhibited by concurrent administration of sodium ipodate. Four groups of rats (mean baseline body weight in each group, 109 g) were injected intraperitoneally once a day with either saline or T_4 (120 µg/day) or ipodate (4 mg/day) or T_4 + ipodate for 11 days. Urine was collected daily in metabolic cages, and urinary urea nitrogen was measured in urine pooled over the duration of the experiment; urinary urea nitrogen values indicated are the average per day for the duration of the experiment. Blood for serum T_4 and T_3 was obtained by decapitation 16 h after the last injection. (Chopra et al. 1978c)

V. Effect of Diet on Serum Concentration of T_3s

Since the BMR drops during fasting and thyroid hormones are important modulators of BMR, changes in circulating thyroid hormone levels during fasting and other dietary changes have received considerable attention recently. As noted above, the serum concentration of T_3 decreases while that of rT_3 increases, and serum T_4 concentration does not change appreciably during complete fasting. These changes in serum T_3 and rT_3 levels become evident within 48 h of initiation of the fast and are maintained for as long as the fast is continued. After 3 or 4 weeks of fasting, however, serum rT_3 decreases and serum T_3 increases toward normal even when the fast is continued (Carlson et al. 1977). Changes in the serum concentration of T_3s similar to those observed during fasting also occur during the administration of hypocaloric diets (Spaulding et al. 1976; Visser et al. 1978a; O'Brian et al. 1978), in protein-calorie malnutrition (Rastogi et al. 1974; Chopra and Smith 1975; Medeiros-Neto et al. 1977), and in anorexia nervosa (Moshang et al. 1975; Miyai et al. 1975, Croxson and Ibbertson 1977).

When an 800-cal diet composed of fat and protein is given to obese subjects, serum T_3 decreases and rT_3 rises in a manner similar to that observed during complete fasting. However, when an 800-cal diet composed only of carbohydrate is administered to obese subjects, no change in T_3 or rT_3 (or T_4) is observed

(Spaulding et al. 1976). These data suggest dietary carbohydrate plays an important role in the maintenance of normal serum T_3 in man. The administration of as few as 200 cal of carbohydrate to human subjects after a 7-day fast or after 14 days of a 400-cal amino acid diet has been shown to restore the low-T_3 and high-rT_3 to normal, even though hypocaloric conditions persisted (O'Brian et al. 1978). Studies in the rat have revealed that, just as in man, serum T_3 falls during fasting (however, serum T_4 also falls during fasting in the rat) and that it returns toward normal within 3 h of refeeding carbohydrate or protein but not fat (Burger et al. 1978). It is possible that the effect of protein administration of T_3 levels of the fasting rat are related to the conversion of protein to glucose via gluconeogenesis.

As opposed to fasting, which is associated with a decrease in oxygen consumption, increased food consumption has been shown associated with an increase in oxygen consumption (Goldman et al. 1975). The effect of excessive caloric consumption on circulating thyroid hormone levels has also been investigated recently (Davidson and Chopra 1979). Six human subjects of normal weight were fed five separate diets; three isocaloric diets (~2000 cal), with 20%, 40%, or 80% carbohydrate, and two hypercaloric (~4000 cal) diets, with 20% or 40% carbohydrate for 5 days; the subjects were fed their usual diets for 1 week between each test diet. Serum T_3, rT_3, and T_4 concentrations were measured on the 6th day of each diet. The mean serum concentrations of T_4 and rT_3 levels after various diets did not differ significantly from one another. However, serum T_3 levels were significantly higher after both hypercaloric diets and the 2000-cal diet containing 80% carbohydrate compared with the 2000-cal diet containing 20% or 40% carbohydrate. Interestingly, however, detailed statistical analysis of the data revealed that the serum T_3 correlates best with total calorie intake ($r = 0.68$, $P<0.001$) rather than with the amount of ingested carbohydrate ($r=0.46$, $P<0.025$), fat ($r=0.49$, $P<0.02$), or protein ($r=0.30$,NS).

These studies clearly suggested an important influence of noncarbohydrate as well as carbohydrate sources of calories on circulating T_3 in man. In addition, these studies made a case that under conditions when at least a normal amount (~200 g) of carbohydrate is ingested, noncarbohydrate sources of calories may influence circulating T_3 to an even greater extent than does carbohydrate (Davidson and Chopra 1979). In other studies, Danforth et al. (1975, 1976) observed significant increases in serum T_3 and decreases in serum rT_3 when human volunteers were fed increased calories given as carbohydrate (up to 500 g/day) for 3 weeks but not as fat (even when given for up to 3 months). However, when metabolic clearance and production rates of T_3 were measured, Danforth and co-workers observed increased values in subjects ingesting excess calories of fat as well as carbohydrate (Danforth E jr, cit. in Chopra et al. 1978c).

The various studies have suggested that increased T_3 production during overeating is due to an alteration (increase) in extrathyroidal conversion of T_4 to T_3 rather than to increased thyroidal secretion. It seems possible that the well-documented increase in oxygen consumption that occurs during overeating (Sims 1976) is related, in part at least, to the concurrent increases in the production rate of T_3. The process of excessive heat generation during excessive food intake has been referred to as "luxuskonsumption" (Goldman et al. 1975; Burse et al. 1977). It may reflect homeostatic mechanism(s) involved in the maintenance of stable body weight.

VI. Effect of Drugs

The serum concentration of T_3s deviates from normal during administration of several pharmacologic agents (Chopra and Solomon 1976). The following discussion applies to agents that alter extrathyroidal metabolism of iodothyronines and deals with changes in iodothyronine levels that occur after the administration of the thyroid hormone preparations, TSH and TRH.

1. Drugs Influencing Extrathyroidal Metabolism of Iodothyronines

Table 4.4 lists a number of drugs which, when administered to hypothyroid subjects being treated with T_4 replacement, are associated with a significant decrease in serum T_3 concentration and a clear increase in serum rT_3 concentration; serum T_4 concentration does not change appreciably after the administration of these drugs (except for agents used for cholecystography which cause an increase in serum T_4 concentration in hypothyroid patients on T_4 replacement therapy). In vitro studies indicate that cholecystography agents and propylthiouracil inhibit T_4 to T_3 conversion by direct interaction with the T_4 5′-monodeiodinase (Chopra 1977; Chopra et al. 1978c; Leonard and Rosenberg 1979). Dexamethasone does not inhibit T_4 to T_3 conversion by rat liver homogenates in vitro, but it has been shown to reduce T_3 production from T_4 in rat liver after in vivo administration (Hufner and Knopfle 1976; Kaplan and Utiger 1978a). In vitro studies also indicate that agents for cholecystography, propylthiouracil as well as dexamethasone, reduce the metabolism of rT_3 (to 3,3′-diiodothyronine), thereby suggesting an explanation for the high serum rT_3 concentration during administration of these drugs. Propranolol, a β-adrenergic blocking agent and Amiodarone, an antiarrhythmic and antianginal agent, have not yet been studied in the manner of other agents listed above; therefore, the mechanisms of their effects on serum levels of T_3s are unknown.

Figure 4.16 presents serum T_3 and rT_3 concentration in athyreotic patients receiving T_4 and in hyperthyroid patients with Graves' disease before and after the administration of dexamethasone, 2 mg every 6 h for 1 day. The serum T_3 concentration dropped about 20% in patients with T_4 replacement and about 40% in Graves' disease patients, whereas serum rT_3 increased 40% and 80%, respectively, in these two groups. Serum T_4 concentration showed no change in hypothyroid patients taking T_4, whereas it decreased about 15% in patients with Graves' disease. When administration of dexamethasone to hyperthyroid patients was continued for up to 5 days, there was no evidence for an escape from its effects on serum T_3 and rT_3 (Fig. 4.17, Chopra et al. 1975c). The T_3-lowering effect of dexamethasone has recently been applied to the treatment of hyperthyroidism. Croxson et al. (1977) noted a 65% fall in serum T_3 within 24 h and an additional 10% decrease during the subsequent 2 days to reach normal levels when hyperthyroid patients were treated with a combination of dexamethasone (2 mg every 6 h), propylthiouracil (150 mg every 6 h), and saturated solution potassium iodide (3 drops every 6 h). Like dexamethasone, administration of glucocorticoids normally produced in vivo, e.g., hydrocortisone and ACTH, is also associated with the lowering of serum T_3 and increase in serum rT_3, but the effects are much less pronounced than those of dexamethasone even when the doses administered are equivalent in terms of

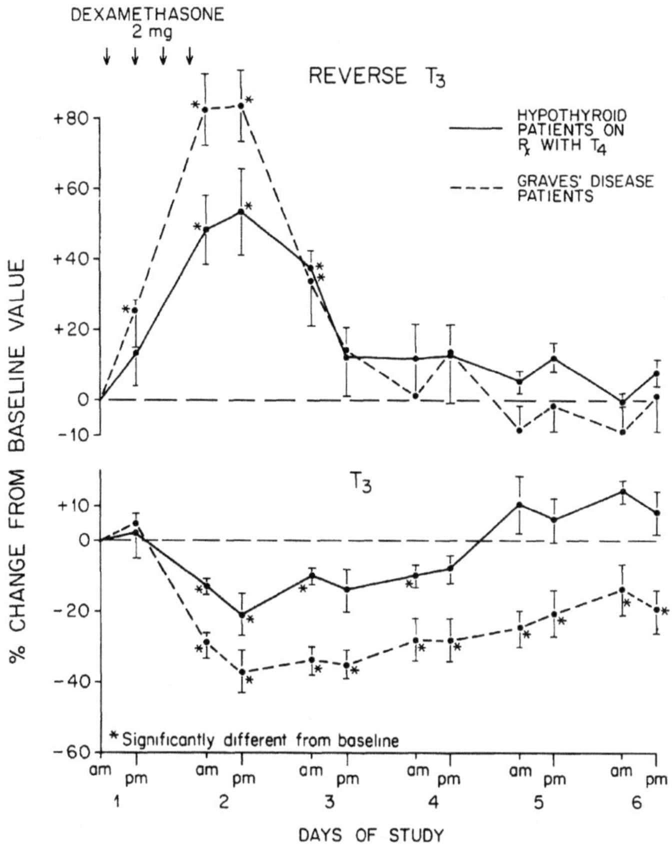

Fig. 4.16. Changes in serum concentration of rT_3 and T_3 following 1 day of administration of dexamethasone (2 mg every 6 h) to hyperthyroid patients with Graves' disease and to hypothyroid patients rendered euthyroid by T_4 replacement. Serum T_4 decreased moderately (~15%) in hyperthyroid patients and did not change appreciably in hypothyroid patients on T_4. Data are expressed as percent change from baseline. (Chopra et al. 1975c)

glucocorticoid effects (Westgren et al. 1977b). The reason for the difference is not known but may be related to the prolonged half-life of dexamethasone.

Sodium ipodate (Oragrafin) is perhaps the most potent radiocontrast agent capable of inhibiting the conversion of T_4 to T_3 by extrathyroidal tissues. The data on serum concentration of iodothyronines following administration of a single oral dose of 3 g sodium ipodate are shown in Fig. 4.18, while those after multiple doses (3 g orally every 3 days) are shown in Fig. 4.19. It is evident that sodium ipodate caused a marked reduction (mean about 75%) in serum T_3 within 48 h of its administration, and the decrease was maintained when sodium ipodate was repeated at 3-day intervals for up to five doses without any evidence of an escape from the effects of the drug (Fig. 4.19). Concomitantly, there was an improvement in hyperthyroidism evidenced by a fall in the pulse rate and pulse pressure and a gain in body weight (Wu et al. 1978b). Whether or not the prompt improvement in the metabolic status of hyperthyroid patients after the administration of sodium ipodate was due merely to the reduction in serum T_3 levels is not clear. It is possible

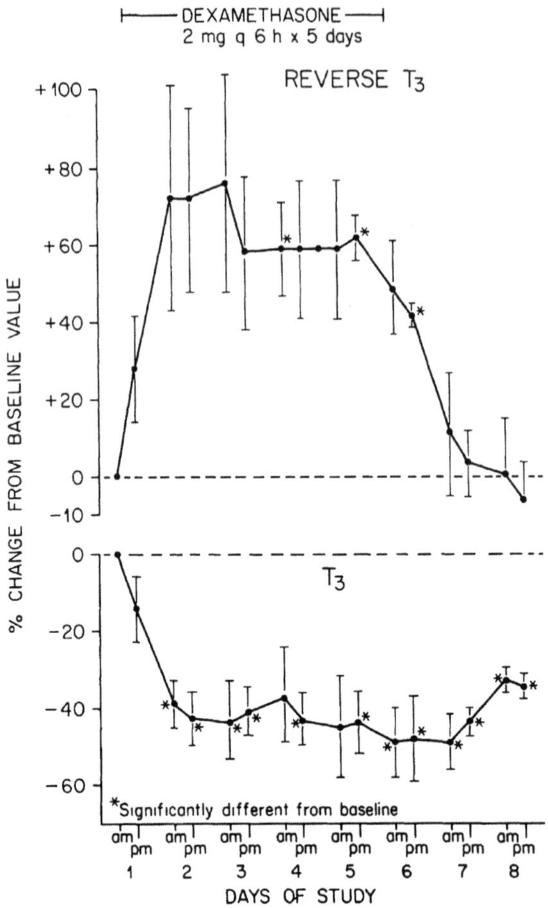

Fig. 4.17. Changes in serum concentrations of rT_3 and T_3 during and following administration of dexamethasone, 2 mg every 6 h for 5 days, to hyperthyroid patients with Graves' disease. Data are expressed as percent change from baseline. (Chopra et al. 1975c)

that in addition to reducing the extrathyroidal conversion of T_4 to T_3, sodium ipodate may also interfere in the binding of thyroid hormones (T_4 to T_3) to cellular (e. g., nuclear) binding sites.

Effects of propylthiouracil, Amiodarone, and propranolol are similar to, but apparently less pronounced than, those of dexamethasone and sodium ipodate described above.

2. Serum Levels of T_3s During Treatment with Thyroid Preparations

Serum concentrations of T_3 and rT_3 are within the normal range and quite stable throughout the day during treatment of hypothyroid patients with replacement doses (0.15–0.2 mg/day) of T_4; serum T_4 levels increase transiently, about 20%–40%, during the first 5 h of T_4 administration (Surks et al. 1972, 1973a). Serum T_4 and rT_3 concentrations are subnormal and stable throughout the day during long-term treatment with T_3. However, serum T_3 levels vary markedly after ingestion of T_3. Serum total T_3 concentrations are maximal at 350–1000 ng/100 ml (upper limit of normal, 210 ng/100 ml) at 2–4 h, while they are normal or slightly high at 24 h after a 50–75 µg/day dose of T_3; the serum concentration of free T_3 is similarly markedly

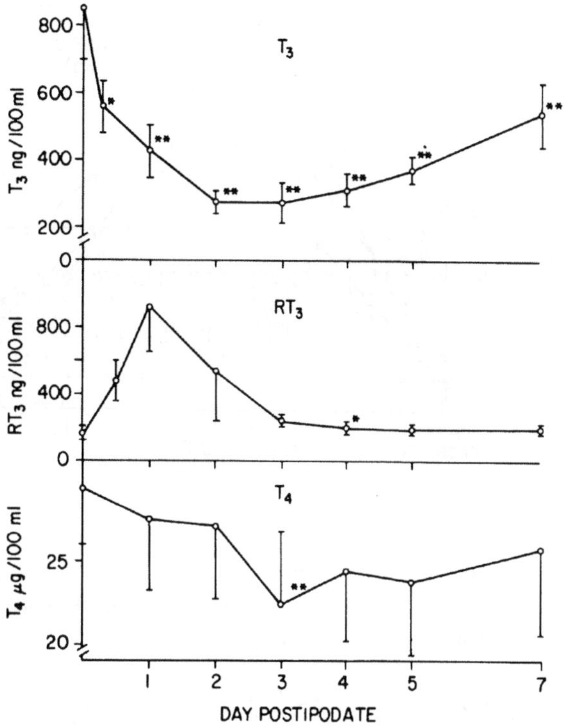

Fig. 4.18. Changes in serum T_3, rT_3, and T_4 after oral administration of 3 g of sodium ipodate to four with hyperthyroid patients Graves' disease. (cf. baseline $* = P < 0.05$; $** = P < 0.01$.) Data are from Wu et al. 1978 a. (Brown et al. 1978)

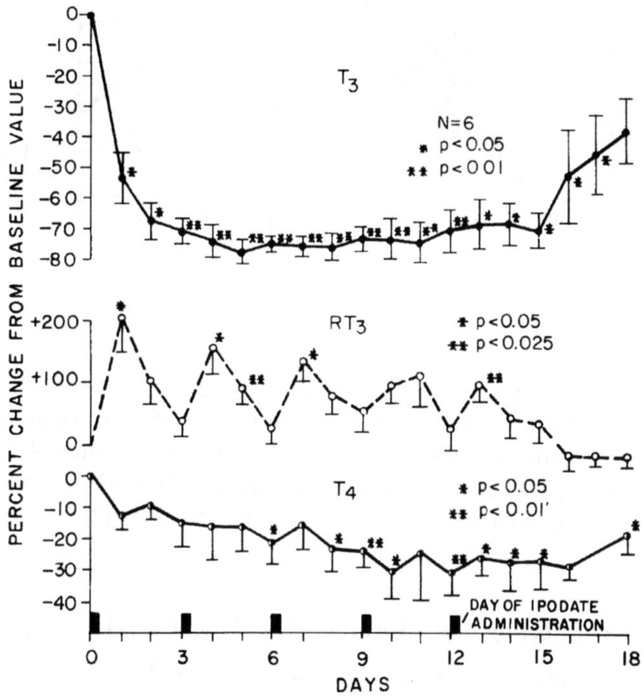

Fig. 4.19. Changes in serum T_3, rT_3, and T_4 in hyperthyroid patients given sodium ipodate, 3 g orally every 3 days for a total of 5 doses). Data are expressed as mean ± S.E.M. of percent changes from baseline value. Data are from Wu et al. 1978 b

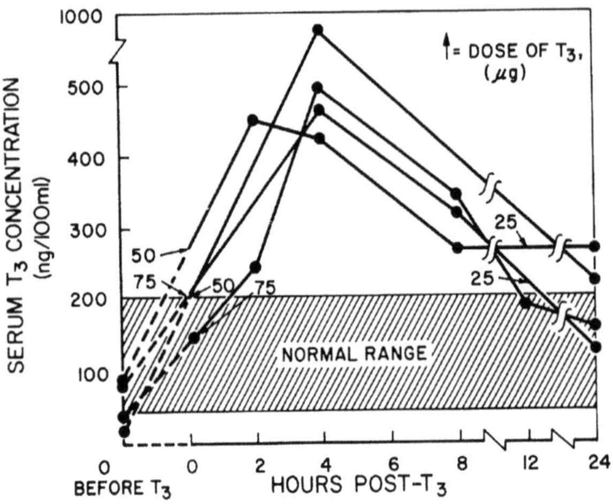

Fig. 4.20. Serum total T_3 concentration in hypothyroid patients before and during oral treatment with T_3. (Chopra et al. 1973 a)

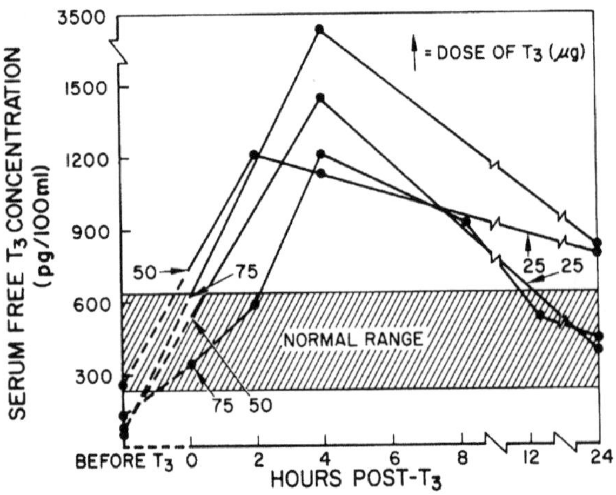

Fig. 4.21. Serum free T_3 concentration in hypothyroid patients before and during oral treatment with T_3. (Chopra et al. 1973 a)

above normal (Figs. 4.20 and 4.21) (Surks et al. 1972; Chopra et al. 1973 a; Kaplan et al. 1977). Serum T_3 levels are two- to fourfold those of normal individuals at 2–8 h, even after the administration of synthetic mixtures of T_4 and T_3 ($T_4 : T_3$, 4 : 1, 180 μg T_4 + 45 μg T_3 per day) or desiccated thyroid (~2 grains/day), and the pattern of change in serum T_3 levels is similar to that after T_3 administration.

3. Effect of Administration of TSH and TRH

The intramuscular injection of 2–10 IU of bovine TSH causes a maximal increase in serum T_3 at about 6 to 8 h and a maximal increase in serum T_4 at about 12–24 h after 10 IU of TSH; the maximal increase above the baseline value approximates 60% (range 36–93) in the case of serum T_4 and about 130% (range 75–195) in the case of

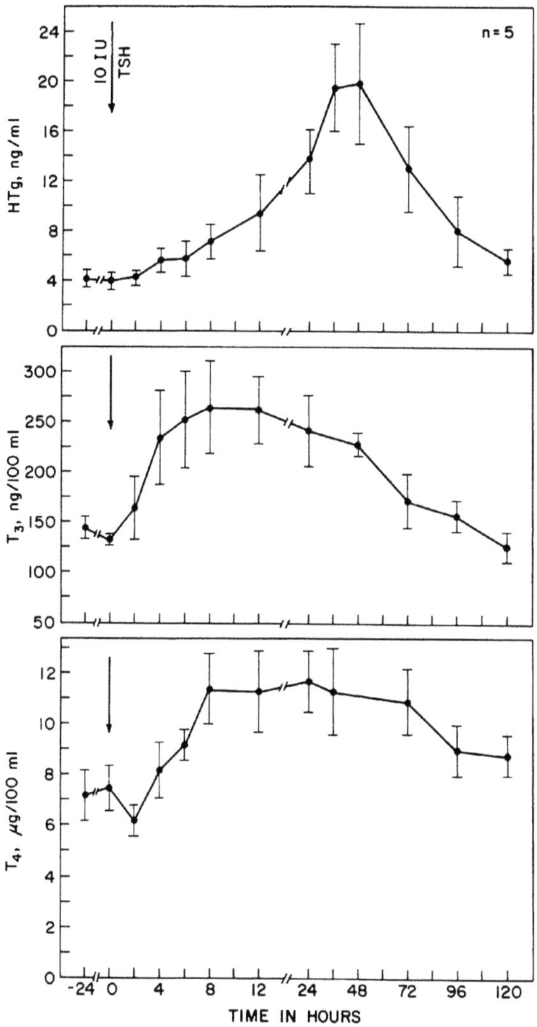

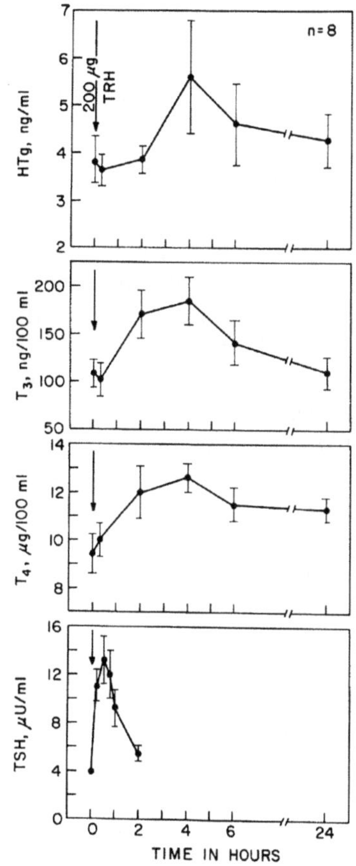

Fig. 4.23

Fig. 4.22

Fig. 4.22. Effect of bovine TSH (Thytropar) on serum thyroglobulin (HTg), T_3, and T_4 concentrations in normal subjects. Data are presented as mean ± S.E. (Uller et al. 1973)

Fig. 4.23. Effect of synthetic thyrotropin-releasing hormone (TRH) on serum thyroglobulin (HTg), T_3, T_4, and TSH concentrations in normal subjects. Data are presented as mean ± S.E. (Uller et al. 1973)

serum T_3 (Fig. 4.22). Serum rT_3 does not change appreciably after intramuscular administration of TSH (Chopra et al. 1972a; Uller et al. 1973; Chopra et al. 1975a).

The intravenous administration of a bolus of synthetic TRH results in an easily measurable increase in serum T_3, a modest increase in serum T_4, and no change in serum rT_3. The maximal increase in serum T_3 and T_4 occurs at 2–4 h (cf. maximal increase in serum TSH at 15–45 min) after intravenous administration of 200 μg of TRH. The mean maximal increase approximates 73% in the case of serum T_3 and 37% in the case of serum T_4 (Fig. 4.23, Chopra et al. 1972a; Uller et al. 1973).

C. Urinary Excretion of T_3s

Urinary T_3 (and T_4) have been measured in several studies from the United Kingdom and Europe, but these measurements have not been popular in the United States. While measurement of urinary T_3 (or T_4) has the advantage of providing an integrated index of thyroid function over many hours or throughout a day, there are several methodologic difficulties. Apparently, salts, urea, and other substances interfere in competitive protein binding assay and to a lesser extent in RIAs used for the measurements. Additionally, urinary excretion of thyroid hormones correlates better with the glomerular filtration rate than with the serum concentration of free thyroid hormones. Even the relationship with glomerular filtration is complicated by tubular excretion and reabsorption of thyroid hormones. While widely varying values of urinary T_3 and T_4 have been noted (Chan et al. 1972; Hufner and Hesch 1973; Shakespeare and Burke 1976; Rogowski et al. 1978), the recent studies utilizing relatively more specific RIA methods of measurement suggest mean normal urinary T_4 and T_3 excretion approximates 1390 and 440 ng/day, respectively ($n=67$). Mean urinary T_4 and T_3 excretion is increased to about twofold and sixfold normal, respectively, in hyperthyroidism, whereas there is a marked reduction to about 10% of normal values in hypothyroidism (Rogowski et al. 1978).

Urinary excretion of rT_3 has also been quantitated recently. Euthyroid individuals excrete about 72 ng rT_3/day, whereas hyperthyroid and hypothyorid patients excrete about 184 and 29 ng/day, respectively. (Faber et al. 1978).

Chapter 5

Kinetics of Peripheral Metabolism and Production Rates of T_3s

A. Methods of Measurement and Normal Values

Conventionally daily production rates (PR) of T_3s are measured by means of disposal rates (DR), which equal PR under steady state conditions. The disposal rate (DR or PR) is calculated by multiplying the serum concentration of iodothyronine (T_3 or rT_3) by its metabolic clearance rate (MCR); MCR refers to the volume of plasma from which iodothyronine is cleared irreversibly per unit time.

Table 5.1 lists several estimates of MCR and the values of T_3s (T_3 and rT_3). The mean normal MCR of T_3 has been estimated to vary between 16 and 27 liters/day, while that of rT_3 has varied between 82 and 131 liters/day. The estimates of mean normal PR of T_3 have varied in recent studies between 23 and 60 μg/day, while those of rT_3 have varied between 21 and 52 μg/day. In comparison, the normal MCR of T_4 has been estimated at about 0.9–1.2 liters/day, while the normal PR of T_4 approximates 90–110 μg/day. The relatively more marked variations in PRs of T_3 and rT_3 reflect the uncertainties in measurement of serum concentration as well as of MCR. The information on the methods of measurement of serum concentration of T_3s has been reviewed in Chap. 4 and that on the measurements of MCRs is discussed below.

In most studies of iodothyronine turnover, a single (pulse) injection of labeled (radioactive) iodothyronine is administered intravenously. The thyroidal uptake of radioactivity is blocked by the oral administration of a saturated solution of potassium iodide, and serial blood samples are obtained at intervals for a few days. The concentration of radioactive iodothyronine at various sampling times is determined and the data are treated mathematically, using one of the several model systems to calculate the rate of disappearance (clearance) of the iodothyronine.

Most of the initial studies employed the single compartment (SC) model for calculating MCR. In this model, it is assumed that iodothyronine is distributed in a single homogeneous and rapidly equilibrating compartment from which it is removed at a constant fractional rate. Using this model, only the terminal slope of the plasma disappearance curve of the labeled iodothyronine is utilized to derive the iodothyronine kinetic parameters. The formulas employed include volume of distribution (VD) = dose divided by zero time intercept of final exponential curve; fractional catabolic rate (FCR) $= 0.693/t\,^1/_2$; MCR = VD × FCR. Unsatisfied by the assumptions of a single compartment model, some investigators employed two or three models, assuming two or three distinct but interconnected compartments, to define the kinetics of iodothyronine distribution (Cavalieri et al. 1970; Koutras et al. 1970). Others employed noncompartmental (NC) techniques for estimation of MCR. One NC technique, which is similar to the method of Tait (1963) used in

Table 5.1. Published data on kinetics of extrathyroidal metabolism of T_3 and reverse T_3

Reference	Serum concen-tration (ng/100ml)	TDV[a] (liters/day)	FCR[a] day	MCR[a] (liters/day)	PR[a] (μg/day)	Mean-resi-dence time (h)[b]	Extra-thyroid-pool (μg/day)	Method of calculation of MCR
T_3								
Sterling et al. 1954	–	–	0.27	–	–	–	–	SC
Wiswell and Coronho 1962	–	–	0.53	–	–	–	–	SC
Fisher and Oddie 1964	–	31.0	0.53	16.4	–	–	–	Whole body counting following single injection
Gregerman and Solomon 1967	–	18.1	0.51	–	–	–	–	SC
Surks and Oppenheimer 1969	–	38.1	0.47	18.0	–	–	–	SC
Woeber et al. 1970	273	43.4	0.52	22.3	60.0	–	–	SC
Cavalieri et al. 1971		35.1	0.75	27.2	–	–	–	SC
		27.8	0.86	26.1				NC following constant influsion
Oddie et al. 1971	97	34.8	0.75	26.1	22.6	–	–	Whole body counting after single injection
Nicoloff et al. 1972	106	36.6	0.68	24.9	26.3	–	–	SC
Inada et al. 1975	142	31.0	0.71	19.8	28.0	–	–	Three compartmental (single injection)
Oppenheimer et al. 1975b,c		21.0	0.72	22.4		–	–	NC (single injection)
Gavin et al. 1977	104	29.3	–	24.0	21.2	–	29.3	NC (single injection)
Suda et al. 1978b	173[c]	–	–	24.0	40.7[a]	–		NC (single injection)
Bianchi et al. 1978	150	27.0	0.98	26.5	41.0	24.7	41.9	NC (single injection)

Reverse T_3								
Chopra, 1976a	48	–	–	81.5	39.5	–	–	NC after single injection of radioactive rT_3
Gavin et al. 1977	32	14.4		104	33	–	4.67	NC after single injection of radioactive rT_3
Smallridge et al. 1978	47	–	–	112	51.7	–	–	NC after single injection of radioactive rT_3
Eisenstein et al. 1978	44 (23)	–	–	96	41.8 (21.4)	–	–	NC after single injection of radioactive rT_3
Suda et al. 1978b	46[c]	–	–	105	49.4[c]	–	–	NC after single injection of radioactive rT_3
Geola et al. 1979	39	–	–	131	44.8	–	–	NC following canstant infusion of radioactive rT_3

[a] TDV = Total distribution volume; FCR = fractional clearance rate; MCR = metabolic clearance rate; PR = production rate. MCR and PR date have been corrected to 70 kg body weight whenever appropriate data were available. SC = Single compartmental; NC = noncompartmental.

[b] Mean residence time = time for which labeled iodothyronine stays, from its release into circulation to its irreversible loss from it.

[c] Studied in subjects taking 0.2 mg/day of T_4, T_4-PR was 140 µg/day.

studies of steroid MCR, employs constant infusion of radioactive T_3 until a stable plasma concentration of labeled T_3 is reached. The rate of infusion of the labeled iodothyronine divided by the equilibrium serum concentration of labeled iodothyronine yields MCR. Another approach in the NC model system is based on measurements of the area under the plasma disappearance curve following a single (pulse) injection of labeled iodothyronine. This NC model system considers a central compartment which is defined as the fast initial distribution space of iodothyronine and includes plasma pool as well as a number of other extravascular pools (compartments) reversibly exchanging the iodothyronine with the central compartment. The term noncompartmental is used for this model system because no definite compartmental localization of iodothyronine is assumed. The MCR is calculated by dividing the dose of labeled iodothyronine administered by the integrated plasma concentration determined by calculating the area under the curve of plasma disappearance curve of the labeled iodothyronine. The reader may refer to Oppenheimer et al. (1975 b, c), Gavin et al. (1977), and Bianchi et al. (1978) for methods of integrating the area under the plasma disappearance curve of iodothyronines.

The published studies comparing SC and NC techniques for determination of MCR regarding T_3 kinetic studies suggest about a 30%–35% overestimation of VD and about a 50% underestimation of FCR by the SC method (Table 5.1, Oppenheimer et al. 1975 b, c; Bianchi et al. 1978). One study found little or no difference in MCRs measured by the two techniques (Cavalieri et al. 1971). However, little or no difference is the usual finding in the studies of MCRs of T_4 by the SC and NC technique (Oppenheimer et al. 1967, 1975 b, c). The greater discrepancy between SC and NC methods of calculation of MCR in cases of T_3 than in those of T_4 may be related to the more rapid fractional removal rate of T_3 in comparison with its rate of distribution. This information served as a guide to using the NC method in most of the recent studies of kinetic parameters of rT_3 (Table 5.1).

Although it offers an improvement over the SC method, the NC method of measuring MCR does have limitations. It does not take into account the iodothyronine molecules (T_3 or rT_3) leaving, but not returning to, the plasma compartment and those that are produced in peripheral tissues but are degraded before ever reaching the plasma compartment. The extent of the effect of such nonexchangeable pools of T_3 or rT_3 on present day estimates of these MCRs is not known.

Another problem in accurate measurement of MCR pertains to the difficulties in appropriate measurement of the concentrations of labeled T_3 (or rT_3) in serum at various time intervals after injection of the label. The metabolism of iodothyronine results in production of radioiodide as well as other radioiodinated products including iodoproteins, less-iodinated iodothyronines (di-and/or monoiodothyronines) and side chain derivatives of iodothyronine (e. g., triiodothyroacetic acid) which must be separated from the radioactivity in the parent (injected) iodothyronine for accurate measurements of its serum concentration. The problem of contamination of T_3 (or T_4) radioactivity with iodoproteins was not recognized until 1969–1970, when Surks and Oppenheimer (1969) employed trichloroacetic acid (TCA) precipitation to remove free iodide followed by ethanol extraction of the precipitate to measure the nonextractable radioactivity in the iodoproteins. The concentration of labeled T_3 (or T_4) was then determined as the difference between the TCA precipitable and the ethanol nonextractable radioactivities. Other workers devised column chromatography methods for separating radioactive T_3 from iodide and iodoproteins (Nicoloff et al. 1972). Rudolph et al. (1978) have recognized a problem in accurately estimating the serum concentration of radioactive iodothyronines that results from contamination of radioactive T_3 and rT_3 in plasma with deiodinative products of their metabolism. Although the effect of radioactive deiodinative metabolites on kinetic studies of T_3 and rT_3 is a relatively modest one compared with that of iodoproteins (Gavin et al. 1977), more recent studies have incorporated appropriate chromatographic steps to take into account their effect (Gavin et al. 1978). Some recent studies have employed specific antibodies in an attempt to determine accurately the concentration of radioactive T_3 and/or rT_3 in plasma for kinetic studies (Aickin et al. 1977; Bianchi et al. 1978). It is hoped that future studies will provide a more precise estimate of the MCRs and PRs of T_3 and rT_3 than are presently available.

B. Alterations in Thyroid Diseases

The MCR of T_3 is increased by about 70%–130% above normal in individuals with hyperthyroidism, whereas it is decreased by about 30% in those with hypothyroidism. There is a good correlation between the MCR of T_3 and serum T_3 concentration when data in all states of thyroid function are analyzed together. It has been suggested that the concentration of free T_3 in serum is an important determinant of T_3 turnover. The mean change in PR-T_3 is about fivefold higher than normal in hyperthyroid patients, whereas it is reduced to 10%–30% of normal in hypothyroidism. These changes in PR-T_3 in hyperthyroid and hypothyroid patients are similar to those seen in free T_3 concentration in hyperthyroidism and hypothyroidism, respectively (Nicoloff et al. 1972; Bianchi et al. 1978).

The MCR of rT_3 is also increased by about 75% above the normal mean value (191 vs. 112 liters/day/70 kg) in hyperthyroidism, whereas it is decreased by about 35% in hypothyroidism. PR-rT_3 is increased to about fivefold higher than normal in hyperthyroidism whereas the values in hypothyroidism average about 10% of normal in hypothyroidism (Smallridge et al. 1978).

The MCR of T_4 averages about 100% above normal in hyperthyroidism whereas values in hypothyroidism show little or no change. PR-T_4 is increased to about three times above normal in hyperthyroidism, and it is reduced to about 20% of normal in hypothyroidism (Nicoloff et al. 1972).

C. Alterations in Nonthyroid Diseases and Low-T_3 Syndrome

The kinetics of metabolism of T_3s have been studied recently in three examples of the low-T_3 syndrome in the adult, namely, hepatic cirrhosis, starvation, and diabetes mellitus. In addition, data have been recorded comparing the fetal and the adult sheep.

The MCR of T_3 does not vary significantly from the normal range in individuals with hepatic cirrhosis (Fig. 5.1) (Nomura et al. 1975; Chopra 1976 a) and in diabetes mellitus (Pittman et al. 1979), whereas both normal and low values have been

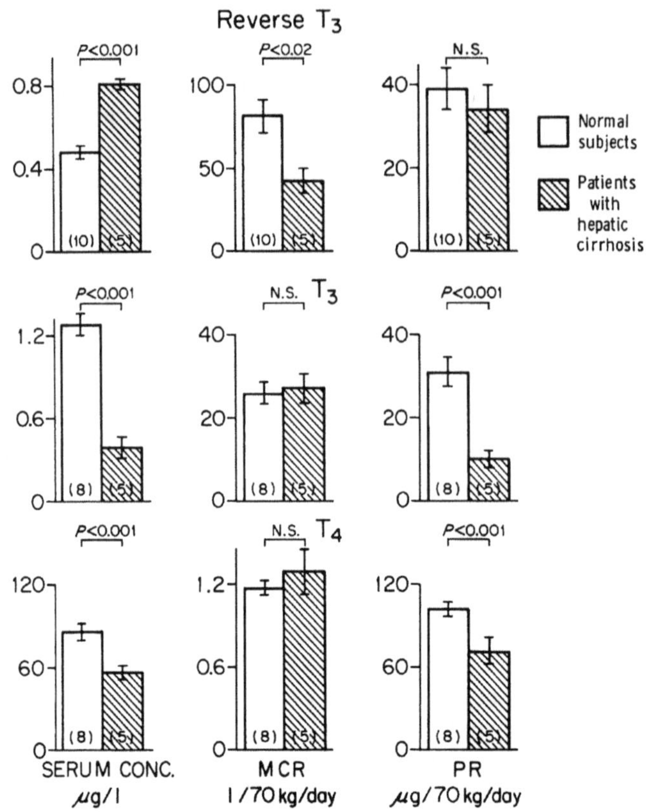

Fig. 5.1. Comparison of serum concentration, MCR, and daily PR of rT_3, T_3, and T_4 in adult patients with hepatic cirrhosis and healthy euthyroid volunteers. Data from Chopra 1976 a. (Chopra et al. 1978 c)

recorded during fasting (Vagenakis et al. 1977; Suda et al. 1978 b). However, as the serum T_3 concentration is clearly reduced, so is the PR-T_3 in each of these three conditions. PR-T_3 is only about 30% of normal in hepatic cirrhosis, in complete fasting, and in insulindependent uncontrolled diabetes mellitus. Since the PR-T_4 is either normal or only modestly reduced (to about 70%–80% of normal) in these conditions, it appears that reduced PR-T_3 in nonthyroid illnesses is caused by a reduced rate of extrathyroidal conversion of T_4 to T_3; this impression has been fortified by several recent studies (Chopra et al. 1975 d; Vagenakis et al. 1975; Chopra 1976 a; Suda et al. 1978 a, b; Pittman et al. 1979).

The MCR of T_3 in fetal sheep is much higher (three- to fourfold) than that in adult sheep. Therefore, even though the serum T_3 concentration is markedly reduced in the fetus, PR-T_3 is similar in both the fetal and the adult sheep. This is the case at a time when fetal PR-T_4 is clearly increased to about twice that of the adult. Since thyroidal content of T_3 and T_4 is similar in the fetus and the adult sheep, a low ratio of PRs of T_3 and T_4 has been explained on the basis of reduced extrathyroidal conversion of T_4 to T_3 (Chopra et al. 1975 b). In vitro studies comparing the ability of T_4 to convert to T_3 in liver and kidney homogenates of fetal and adult sheep have supported this inference (Wu et al. 1978 c).

The MCR of rT_3 has been reduced in all four of the above-mentioned instances of low-T_3 syndrome which have been studied so far. It is reduced by about 50% in hepatic cirrhosis, by about 30%–50% in complete fasting and only about 8%–10% in diabetes mellitus. MCR-rT_3 is markedly reduced (by about 70%) in the fetal sheep compared with the adult. Since the serum concentration of rT_3 is increased, PR-rT_3 remains normal in hepatic cirrhosis (Fig. 5.1), in fasting, and in diabetes mellitus. However, it is clearly higher in fetal sheep than in the adult, apparently because PR-T_4, and consequently the substrate for rT_3 production, is increased in the fetus (Fig. 4.3). The ratio of PRs of rT_3 and T_4 (rT_3/T_4) is either normal or moderately increased in all of the above-mentioned situations including the fetus (Chopra et al. 1975 b; Chopra 1976 a; Eisenstein et al. 1978; Suda et al. 1978 a, b; Pittman et al. 1979).

Chapter 6

Sources of T_3s: Thyroidal Secretion Versus Extrathyroidal Metabolism of T_4

In determining the sources of circulating T_3, the description of the pathway for the conversion of T_4 to T_3 (Pitt-Rivers et al. 1955) and its confirmation in man (Braverman et al. 1970; Pittman et al. 1971) as well as in animal species (Schwartz et al. 1971; Fisher et al. 1972) led to the question of the relative significance of extrathyroidal metabolism versus thyroidal secretion. This question was important because its answer reflects on the extent to which T_4 is normally metabolized by conversion to T_3 and the extent to which the metabolic activity of T_4 may depend on its conversion to a metabolically more potent T_3. Subsequently, when the existence of rT_3 in human circulation and thyroglobulin became known, and when it was realized that, as in the case of T_3, the peripheral metabolism of T_4 is also an important source of rT_3, questions were raised about the relative significance of thyroidal secretion versus extrathyroidal metabolism of T_4 as sources of rT_3. Answers to these were important to help understand more fully the relative importance in health (and subsequently in disease) of the pathway of inner ring monodeiodination of T_4 compared with the outer ring monodeiodination to T_3 (Chopra 1974, 1976 a).

A simple approach to the assessment of the significance of thyroidal secretion of T_3s depends on the estimation of relative proportions of T_3 (or rT_3) and T_4 in thyroglobulin, followed by multiplication of the T_3/T_4 (or rT_3/T_4) ratio in thyroglobulin by the daily PR-T_4. Recent estimates of the T_3/T_4 ratio in human thyroglobulin have varied between 0.051 and 0.096 (Nagataki et al. 1972; Chopra et al. 1973 b; Larsen et al. 1973), whereas those of the rT_3/T_4 ratio have varied between 0.013 and 0.047 (Chopra 1974, 1976 a; Burman et al. 1977 b). Multiplying these values with a PR-T_4 of about 90 µg/day (Van Middlesworth 1974), the thyroid secretion rate (TSR) may be calculated to vary between 4.6 and 8.4 µg/day for T_3 and between 1.2 and 4.2 g/day for rT_3; these estimates represent only a minor fraction of PR-T_3 and PR-rT_3, respectively (Table 5.1). The superiority of this approach for estimating TSR is that it does not have to depend on the data of the serum concentration and MCR of T_3 and rT_3, which have varied over a wide range in different studies (Chap. 4). The basic assumptions in this method consider that (1) thyroidal secretion is the only source of T_4; (2) PR-T_4 can be measured reliably; (3) T_3 (or rT_3) and T_4 are secreted in the proportion in which they exist in thyroglobulin. The first two assumptions are probably valid, although the third one may be questioned. There are data that suggest a preferential secretion of T_3 in the rat (Haibach 1971), as well as rT_3 in the dog (Laurberg 1978). On the other hand, other studies have suggested a good agreement between the T_3/T_4 ratio in thyroidal secretory products and in thyroglobulin (Abrams and Larsen 1973). Unfortunately, at the present time similar data are not available for man. However, studies indicating a nearly normal serum concentration as well as daily production of T_3 (Surks et al. 1973 a) and rT_3 (Chopra 1974; Gavin et al. 1977) in hypothyroid patients receiving replacement therapy with T_4 indicate that extrathyroidal metabolism of T_4 is the major source of both T_3 as well as rT_3 in the circulation of man. A similar conclusion has been drawn from the results of turnover studies in man.

In the normal man, T_4 is mainly metabolized by the process of deiodination. Deiodination has been shown to affect as much as 85% of T_4 produced daily (Berson and Yalow 1954; Ingbar and Freinkel 1955; Oddie et al. 1964). Recent studies suggest that 77%–89% of PR-T_4 may be accounted for by monodeiodinative conversion to T_3 or rT_3 (Chopra 1976 a; Gavin et al. 1977; Suda et al. 1978 b). The amount of T_4 converted to rT_3 was higher than that converted to T_3 in each of these studies, suggesting that inner ring deiodination of T_4 may normally be a more active pathway than the outer ring deiodination to T_3.

Besides being deiodinated, T_4 may also be metabolized by deamination and decarboxylation to TETRAC (Braverman et al. 1970). The data on serum concentration and kinetics of the peripheral metabolism of tetraiodothyroacetic acid (TETRAC) suggest that conversion to TETRAC is only a minor pathway of metabolism of T_4; calculations from the available data suggest that normal PR-TETRAC may only be 3 µg/day or about 4% of PR-T_4 (Chopra et al. 1978 c). In addition to the above-mentioned routes of metabolism T_4 may also be disposed in bile or urine as T_4 or T_4 conjugates. These routes of disposal of T_4 have been estimated to account for about 15% of PR-T_4 (Fig. 6.1).

The data on the effect of various (thyroidal or nonthyroidal) disease states on routes of metabolism are incomplete. There is essentially no direct information on the effect on nondeiodinative pathways of metabolism of T_4, whereas only one of the two deiodinative routes (i. e., conversion to T_3 or rT_3) of metabolism of T_4 has been studied in several diseases.

Recent studies suggest that peripheral conversion of T_4 to T_3 is increased in both hyperthyroidism and hypothyroidism and that there is a fall toward normal after treatment of both disorders. Thus, the T_4 to T_3 conversion rate in hyperthyroid patients dropped in the study of Maguire et al. (1976) from a mean value of 58% to 37% at 3 months to 2 years after treatment of hyperthyroidism. Similarly, they observed a fall in the conversion rate in hypothyroid patients from a mean value of 61% to 44% after treatment with replacement doses (0.15–0.2 mg/day) of T_4 for 9 months to 2 years. Inada et al. (1975) have also recorded a 40% above normal rate of conversion of T_4 to T_3 in hypothyroidism. Little information is available at present on the effect of thyroid disease on the rate of conversion of T_4 to rT_3.

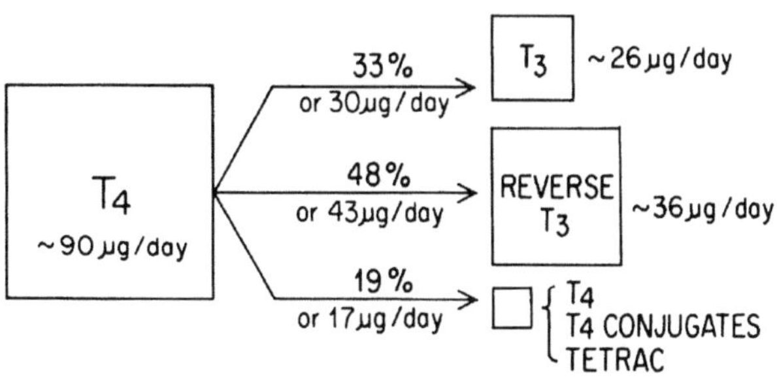

Fig. 6.1. Estimates of the relative magnitude of various routes of metabolism of T_4. (Adapted from Chopra 1976 a)

Alterations in the deiodination of T_4 to T_3 and to rT_3 have been directly examined simultaneously in two examples of the low-T_3 syndrome in adult patients, i. e., complete fasting and diabetes mellitus, while indirect assessment has been made in patients with hepatic cirrhosis. In complete fasting, the rate of conversion of T_4 to T_3 was reduced by about 50% (17% vs. 35%), whereas the rate of conversion of T_4 to rT_3 was increased by about 50% (61% vs. 42%) (Suda et al. 1978 b). Similarly, the T_4 to T_3 conversion rate was found reduced in diabetes mellitus, more so in insulin-dependent (7% vs. 35%) than in insulin-independent (15%) patients. However, the rate of conversion of T_4 to rT_3 was also somewaht lower in diabetic patients than in normal subjects (25% in insulin-dependent and 30% in insulin-independent patients versus 42% in normal subjects). Whereas the amount of T_4 metabolized via conversion to T_3 and rT_3 (76% vs. 77%) in fasting did not differ from normal, it was reduced considerably (45% vs. 77%) in patients with diabetes mellitus. Treatment of diabetic patients with insulin for 2 weeks led to an increase in the T_4 to T_3 conversion rate and a decrease in T_4 to rT_3 conversion rate toward normal, but the amount of T_4 converted to T_3 and rT_3 remained essentially unchanged at 48%. These data suggest that above normal quantities of T_4 are diverted to nondeiodinative routes of metabolism in diabetic patients (Pittman et al. 1979).

The changes in deiodinative routes of metabolism of T_4 in patients with hepatic cirrhosis were similar to those who underwent complete fasting. Thus, there was a clear decrease in the conversion of T_4 to T_3; that to rT_3 was either clearly normal or moderately increased. The overall rate of deiodination of T_4 was slightly less in patients with hepatic cirrhosis (72% vs. 84%) than in normal subjects (Chopra 1976 a).

Chapter 7

Nature of the Processes of and Factors Influencing Production of T_3s from T_4

A. Outer-Ring Monodeiodination of T_4 to T_3

A systematic examination of the mechanism of the outer ring or 5′-monodeiodination of T_4 to T_3 in vitro started with the studies of Albright, Larson, and their co-workers (Albright et al. 1954; Albright and Larson 1959) who demonstrated clear evidence for the conversion in kidney slices and suggested that the process is enzymic in nature. However, these observations stimulated limited interest in the area, probably because the existence of conversion T_4 to T_3 in vivo was questioned (Lassiter and Stanbury 1958). After redemonstration of the process in man (Braverman et al. 1970), there has been an impressive resurgence of interest in the in vitro studies.

The conversion of T_4 to T_3 has now been demonstrated in several human and animal tissues including liver, kidney, heart, fibroblasts, and peripheral blood leukocytes (Sterling et al. 1972; Refetoff et al. 1972; Woeber and Ingbar 1973; Hesch et al. 1975; Green 1976; Visser et al. 1976, 1978 b; Chiraseveenprapund et al. 1976, 1978; Chopra 1977). The question of its occurrence in pituitary tissue has also been addressed, but the results have been controversial. Some researchers have demonstrated the phenomenon using normal human and rat pituitaries as well as the mouse thyrotropic tumors (Grinberg et al. 1963; Volpert et al. 1962) whereas others studying rat pituitary were either unable to find T_3 production from T_4 (Galton 1976) or found T_3 in very small quantities (Chopra et al. 1978 b). More recently, Silva and Larsen (1977) and Silva et al. (1978) have provided new evidence indicating that T_4 to T_3 conversion occurs in vivo in the rat and that T_3 produced locally in the pituitary represents an important fraction (40%–50%) of T_3 bound to pituitary nuclear receptors.

The finding of T_4 to T_3 conversion in many organ systems raises the question of the relative importance of various organs in contributing to the daily production rate of T_3. In vitro studies suggest that on a per gram basis, the liver and kidney are the more potent converters of T_4 to T_3 than various other tissues (Fig. 7.1). However, this information is not sufficient for a clear explanation for T_3 production. It is possible that large organs, e. g., skeletal muscles, contribute importantly to overall T_3 production even though their ability to convert T_4 to T_3 on a per gram weight basis is much lower than that of the liver or kidney.

The detailed studies of T_4 to T_3 converting activity have been conducted using rat liver or kidney homogenates. The data indicate that T_3 generation from T_4 is influenced by factors such as tissue and substrate (T_4) concentration, pH, temperature, and the duration of incubation. The dependence of T_4 to T_3 converting activity on temperature (optimal at 37° C), on pH (optimal at 6–7), as

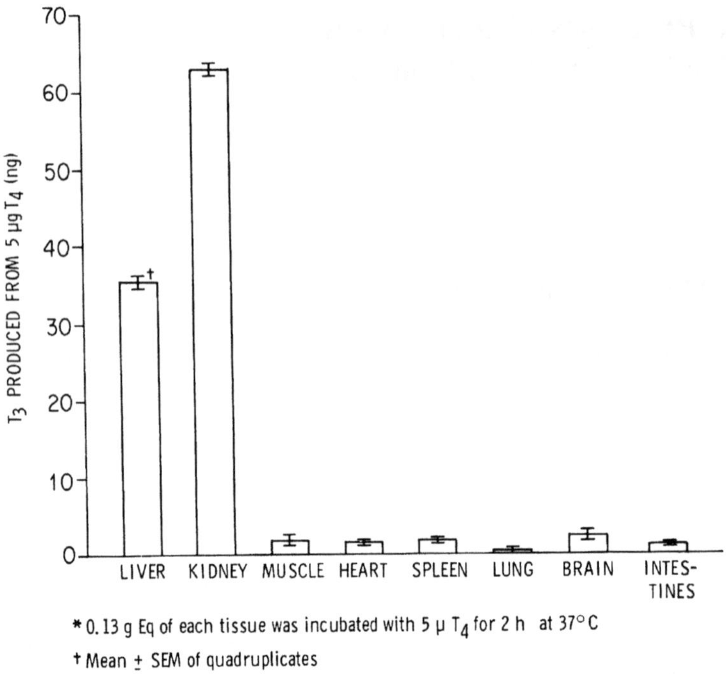

Fig. 7.1. Comparison of the relative potency of conversion of T_4 to T_3 by homogenates of various rat tissues. Data from Chopra 1977. (Chopra et al. 1978c)

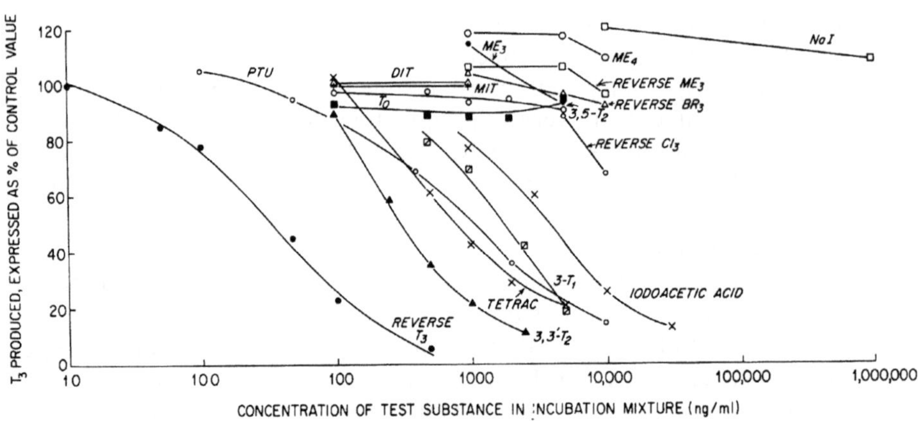

Fig. 7.2. Comparison of the effect of several thyroid analogues, propylthiouracil (PTU), and iodoacetic acid on conversion of T_4 to T_3 by rat liver homogenate in vitro. Approximately 130 mg-equivalent tissue homogenates in 0.15 *M* phosphate buffer (pH 7.3) were incubated with 5 μg of T_4 for 2 h at 37° C, and the T_3 generated was quantified by RIA of an ethanol extract of incubation mixture. The amount of T_3 produced in control tubes, i.e., tubes containing tissue and T_4 without any test agents, was arbitrarily assigned a value of 100 and that produced in the presence of test agents was expressed as percentage of control tubes. TETRAC = tetraiodothyroacetic acid; 3,3'-T_2 = 3,3'-diiodothyronine; 3-T_1 = 3-monoiodothyronine; MIT = monoiodothyrosine; DIT = diiodothyrosine; To = L-thyronine; 3,5-T_2 = 3,5-diiodothyronine; ME_3 = methylated analogue of T_3; ME_4 = methylated analgue of T_4; reverse ME_3 = methylated analgue of rT_3; reverse BR_3 = brominated analog up of rT_3; reverse CL_3 = chlorinated analogue of rT_3; NaI = sodium iodide. (Chopra et al. 1978c)

well as its heat lability strongly suggest that it is enzymic in nature (Chopra 1977; Hufner et al. 1977; Visser et al. 1978 b). Cell fractionation studies of the rat liver and kidney suggest that the activity is located predominantly in the particulate fractions of the cell. It appears to reside predominantly in the plasma membranes and microsomes of the kidney (Leonard and Rosenberg 1978) and liver (Maciel et al. 1979). The apparent Km of rat liver and kidney homogenates and sheep liver homogenates for T_4 to T_3 conversion activity has measured between 1 and 5 μM in various studies. The converting activity is uninfluenced by large doses of iodide, monoiodotyrosine, diiodotyrosine, 3,5-T_2, methylated, brominated, or chlorinated T_3 and rT_3 (Fig. 7.2), and methimazole. It is inhibited in a dose-dependent manner

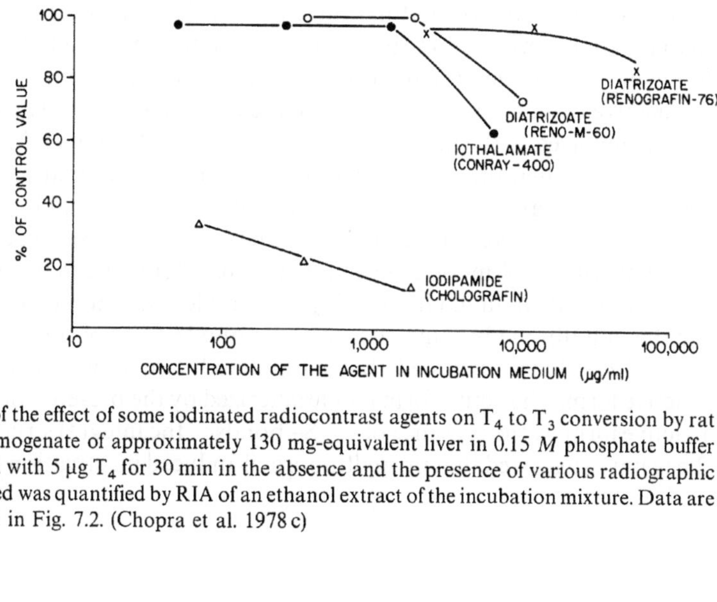

Fig. 7.3. Comparison of the effect of some iodinated radiocontrast agents on T_4 to T_3 conversion by rat liver homogenate. Homogenate of approximately 130 mg-equivalent liver in 0.15 *M* phosphate buffer (pH 7.3) was incubated with 5 μg T_4 for 30 min in the absence and the presence of various radiographic agents. The T_3 produced was quantified by RIA of an ethanol extract of the incubation mixture. Data are expressed as described in Fig. 7.2. (Chopra et al. 1978 c)

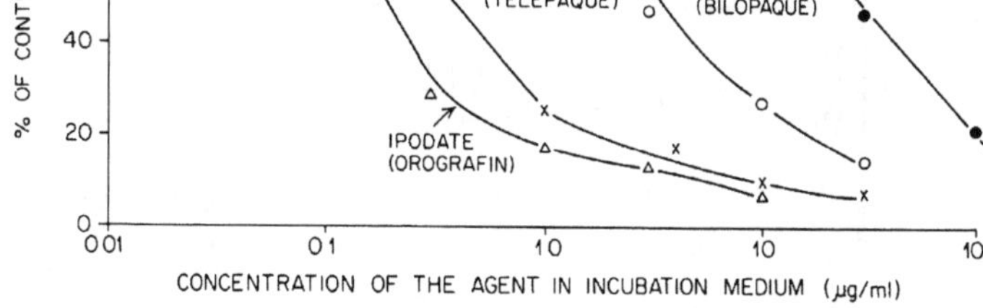

Fig. 7.4. Comparison of the effect of various radiographic agents used for cholecystography on T_4 to T_3 conversion by rat liver homogenate. The experimental design and the method of expression of results are described in Fig. 7.3. (Chopra et al. 1978 c)

by rT_3, $3',5'-T_2$, TETRAC, $3,3'-T_2$, propylthiouracil, iodoacetic acid and by iodinated radiocontrast agents used for oral cholecystography (Figs. 7.3, 7.4). Reverse T_3, $3',5'-T_2$, and sodium ipodate used for oral cholecystography are similar in potency and inhibit the T_4 to T_3 conversion in a competitive manner; their Ki (Michaelis Constant of the Inhibitor) approximates 0.045, 0.041, and 0.038 μM, respectively. The nature of the inhibitory effect of TETRAC and $3,3'T_2$ on conversion of T_4 to T_3 has not yet been determined. Iodoacetic acid is a noncompetitive inhibitor, whereas propylthiouracil is an uncompetitive inhibitor of T_4 to T_3 conversion activity (Chopra 1977; Chopra et al. 1978 c).

Sulfhydryl groups are vital to the ability of tissues to convert T_4 to T_3. Thus, thiol agents, e.g., dithiothreiotol (DTT), mercaptoethanol, and reduced glutathione stimulate the process, whereas SH-oxidizing reagents, diamide, SH-binding reagents, *N*-ethylmaleimide, and mercuric chloride, as well as oxidized glutathione inhibit T_4 to T_3 monodeiodination (Fig. 7.5). The chemical mechanisms by which SH groups are involved in the monodeiodination may include one or both of the following possibilities: (1) the conformation of monodeiodinase may be altered from an inactive to an active site because of the participation of SH groups at or close to the site involved in the monodeiodination of T_4 to T_3, and (2) SH groups may serve as cofactors when the enzyme catalyzes the monodeiodination of T_4 to T_3. Some recent studies have favored the first possibility (Leonard and Rosenberg 1978, 1979; Yamada et al. 1978). The studies of Yamada et al. (1978) suggest that glutathione interacts with T_4 5'-monodeiodinase at a site different from the one that reacts with T_4, and propylthiouracil inhibits T_4 5'-monodeiodination by its ability to compete for the glutathione binding site on the monodeiodinase. Leonard and Rosenberg (1978, 1979) have suggested that monodeiodinase is present in an active and an inactive form. The active form is characterized by the presence of SH groups and the inactive form by the presence of –S–S– bonds in the integral structure of the enzyme. They have suggested that propylthiouracil-induced inactivation of monodeiodinase

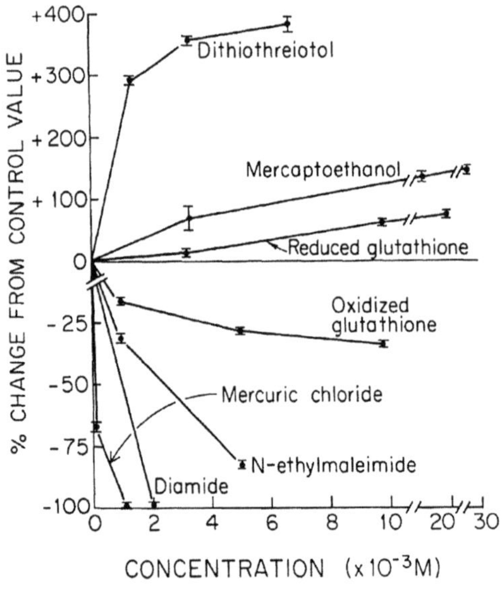

Fig. 7.5. Effect of sulfhydryl reagents on conversion of T_4 to T_3 by rat liver homogenate. Chopra IJ (1978) Sulfhydryl groups and the monodeiodination of thyroxine to triiodothyronine. Science 199: 904–906. Copyright by the American Association for the Advancement of Science

is related to the binding of propylthiouracil with enzyme disulfide groups (Leonard and Rosenberg 1979).

In addition to the SH groups, nicotinamide adenine dinucleotide phosphate (NADPH or TPNH) has also been implicated as an important stimulator of T_4 to T_3 conversion (Balsam and Ingbar 1978 a). However, NADPH (or the NADPH-regenerating system) does not stimulate the conversion in the absence of thiol agents, suggesting that it may be involved secondarily either by stimulating the regeneration of SH groups (as glutathione) (Fig. 7.6) or by reducing their oxidation.

The information suggesting an important influence of tissue SH groups on enzymic conversion of T_4 to T_3 has prompted studies of the role of changes in their tissue concentration in the reduced conversion of T_4 to T_3 in some situations, e. g., fetal life and complete fasting. Some pertinent information is reviewed below.

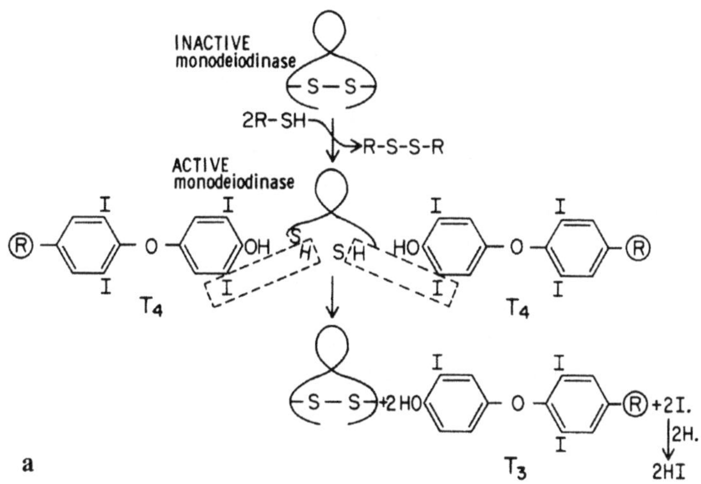

a

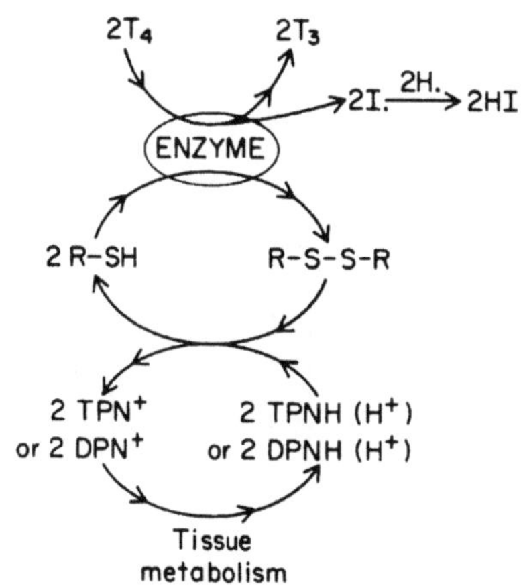

b

Fig. 7.6 a, b. Some mechanisms by which sulfhydryl groups may influence outer-ring monodeiodination of T_4. **a** Sulfhydryl groups alter conformation of enzyme to an active form. **b** Sulfhydryl groups act as cofactor, and enzyme itself is unchanged. Both mechanisms may also be involved. (Chopra et al. 1978 c)

That fetal tissues generate, on a per unit weight basis, much less T_3 than adult tissues has been shown in the sheep, the rat, and the rabbit (Chopra 1978 b; Wu et al. 1978 b; Harris et al. 1978, 1979; Segall-Blank 1978). This characteristic of fetal tissues changes shortly after birth. The newborn sheep tissue homogenates generate T_3 from T_4 as well as or better than adult sheep tissues within 2–8 h after birth (Wu et al. 1978 c). Interestingly, when fetal tissues are incubated with T_4 in the presence of a thiol protective agent, DTT, the amount of T_3 generated is similar to or greater than that generated when T_4 is incubated with adult sheep tissues in the presence of DTT (Fig. 7.7). These data suggest that the main reason for reduced T_4 to T_3 conversion by fetal sheep tissues compared with adult sheep tissues may be the decreased availability of SH groups rather than the deficiency of T_4 5'-monodeiodinase. This inference is supported by the data on the hepatic concentration of nonprotein (free) SH groups. Thus, the hepatic concentration of free SH groups is much lower in the fetal sheep than in adult sheep, whereas that in the neonatal liver is similar to that in the adult und much greater than that in the fetus (Fig. 7.8; Chopra 1978 b). As in the case of fetal sheep, T_4 to T_3 converting activity, as well as free SH group concentration in liver homogenates, is clearly lower in the fetal rat than in the adult rat. However, normalization of these parameters does not occur until 5–7 day of postnatal life (cf. 2–8 h in sheep). Harris et al. (1978, 1979) have proposed that low T_4 to T_3 converting activity in the fetal rat liver is due to a combination of a decrease in SH groups and a decrease in the concentration of the deiodinase. Studies in the rabbit have suggested that the low T_3 generating ability of fetal liver results from a combination of reduced concentration of available SH groups and a reduced affinity of the monodeiodinase for T_4 (Segall-Blank 1978).

A reduction in T_3 generating ability of tissues during fasting has been documented in several studies of liver homogenates (and or slices) of rats starved for 2–4 days (Kaplan and Utiger 1978 a; Balsam et al. 1977; Balsam and Ingbar 1978 a, b; Harris et al. 1978; Chopra and Solomon 1979). The addition of thiol agent, DTT,

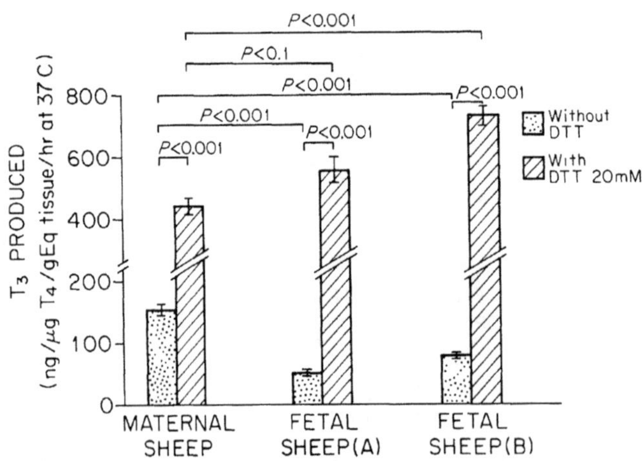

Fig. 7.7. Comparison of the effect of a thiol protective agent, dithiothreitol (DTT), on T_4 to T_3 converting ability of liver homogenates of adult sheep and fetal sheep of 135 days' gestation (term in sheep is ~140–145 days). Data are from Chopra 1978 b. (Chopra et al. 1978 c)

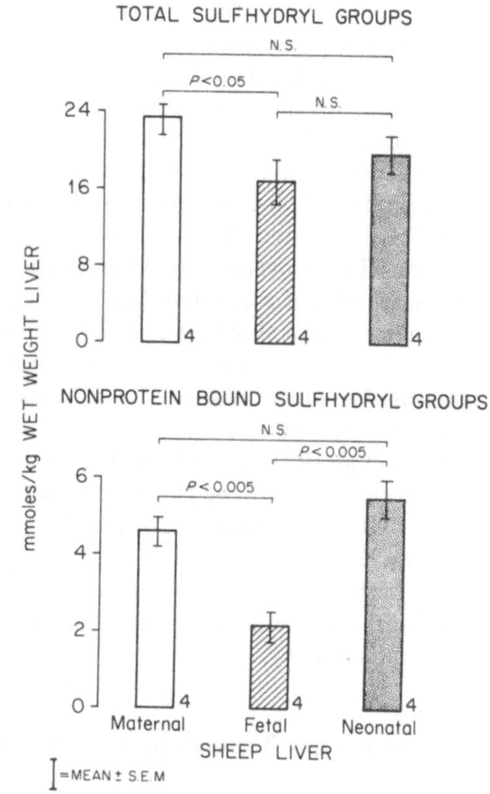

Fig. 7.8. Comparison of the concentration of total and nonprotein bound (free) sulfhydryl groups in liver homogenates of maternal, fetal, and neonatal sheep. Data are from Chopra 1978 b. (Chopra et al. 1978 c)

restores the T_3 generating ability of liver homogenates of rats fasted for 2 days but not of those fasted for 4 days. The hepatic concentration of nonprotein SH groups (NP-SH) is reduced at 2 days but tends to increase toward normal by 4 days, presumably because of an increased availability, from increased protein metab olism, of sulfur-containing amino acids for glutathione synthesis. When rats are treated with T_4 during starvation, the T_4 to T_3 converting activity in liver homogenates is subnormal at 2 days when the concentration of available NP-SH groups is low, but it is restored toward normal at 4 days when the hepatic concentration of free SH groups improves (Chopra and Solomon 1979). These data, and those indicating that (1) serum concentration of thyroid hormones is subnormal at 4 days of starvation (Kaplan and Utiger 1978 a, b; Chopra et al. 1978 b) and (2) hypothyroidism in associated with a reduction in T_3-generating ability of rat tissues (Balsam et al. 1977; Harris et al. 1979), suggest that reduced T_4 to T_3 converting activity in liver of a starved rat is due to a reduction in free SH groups initially and subsequently mainly to hypothyroidism (Chopra and Solomon 1979). Starvation, even when prolonged for several weeks, is not associated with hypothyroidism in man (Portnay et al. 1974; Carlson et al. 1977). Furthermore, hypothyroidism is associated with an increase (rather than a decrease noted in the rat) in the rate of extrathyroidal conversion of T_4 to T_3 in man (Inada et al. 1975; Maguire et al. 1976). Therefore, it is conceivable that a reduction in hepatic free SH groups is the main factor responsible for the reduced T_4 to T_3 conversion in the tissues of fasting man. In this respect, it is interesting to recall that characteristically low serum T_3 and high serum rT_3 resulting from alterations in peripheral metabolism of iodothyronines in fasting humans tend to improve toward normal after the second week of fasting (Carlson et al. 1977; Suda et al. 1978 b). This improvement may be related to a gradual increase in tissue concentration of free SH groups during prolonged fasting.

The finding of variable amounts of T_4 to T_3 converting activity in various tissues (Fig. 7.1) has raised the question of whether identical or different isozymes are involved. The converting activities in rat liver and kidney homogenates are quite similar in terms of optimal pH (6.0–7.0), Km for conversion (1–5 μM), stimulation by thiol agents, and inhibition by propylthiouracil, SH-oxidizing (or binding) agents, and radiocontrast agents, e. g., sodium ipodate. They are similar, but not identical, in terms of a reduction in activity during starvation and hypothyroidism; the effects of these situations are much more marked in liver than in kidney homogenates (Balsam et al. 1977; Balsam and Ingbar 1978 a; Ferguson et al. 1979). The T_4 to T_3 converting activity in the pituitary gland, however, differs from that in liver in some respects. Thus, hypothyroidism and hyperthyroidism stimulate and inhibit, respectively, the T_4 to T_3 converting activity in the pituitary, whereas they have opposite effects in the liver (Kaplan 1978). Therefore, the possibility cannot be ruled out that the T_4 5′-monodeiodinase in the pituitary may be different from that in the liver or the kidney.

B. Inner-Ring Monodeiodination of T_4 to Reverse T_3

Study of the conversion phenomenon of T_4 to rT_3 has been difficult in vitro because rT_3 is rapidly further metabolized in the outer-ring to 3,3′-T_2. Inner-ring monodeiodination of T_4 to rT_3 has, however, been demonstrated in monkey hepatocarcinoma cells, which are deficient in their ability to deiodinate iodothyronines in the outer ring (Sorimachi and Robbins 1977). Grussendorf et al. (1977) first demonstrated the conversion of T_4 to rT_3 by homogenates of normal rat liver at pH 9.5; this high pH inhibits the degradation of rT_3. Cavalieri et al. (1977) studied the conversion of T_4 to rT_3 using cytosol from the rat liver, which also is very weak compared with the whole homogenate, in degrading rT_3 (or T_4) in the outer- ring. Visser et al. (1978 b) estimated the properties of the T_4 to rT_3 conversion system in the rat liver homogenate by studying the conversion of T_4 to 3,3′-T_2; their method of study may be suboptimal because of the error introduced by 3,3′-T_2 generated from metabolism of T_3 that is produced concurrently with rT_3 during incubation of the rat liver homogenate with T_4. However, the error is probably not large because the conversion rate of T_3 to 3,3′-T_2 in the liver homogenate is much slower than that of rT_3 to 3,3′-T_2 (Chopra et al. 1978 a).

Like T_4 to T_3 converting activity, T_4 to rT_3 converting activity is also enzymic in nature (Cavalieri et al. 1977); its Km has been estimated at about 5 μM; its optimal pH is 8.0–8.2, and its optimal temperature is 37° C. The aspects of its dependence on available SH groups, inactivation by heat, and inhibition by propylthiouracil are also similar to those of T_4 to T_3 converting activity. Similarly, methimazole and the lack of light or oxygen have no inhibitory effect on the conversion of T_4 to rT_3 or T_3. However, an optimal pH of 8.0–8.2 (instead of 6.0–7.0 for T_4 to T_3 converting activity) (Cavalieri et al. 1977; Visser et al. 1978 b) and an abundance of T_4 to rT_3 converting activity in the rat liver cytosol (instead of particlate fractions) suggest that the monodeiodinases deiodinating T_4 in the inner-ring (to rT_3) and in the outer-ring (to T_3) are distinct from each other. Studies with purified preparations of the enzyme(s) should provide the definitive information in this regard.

Chapter 8

Routes of T_3s Metabolism

A. In Vivo Studies

Recent studies suggest that, as in the case of T_4, monodeiodination (to T_2s) is an important mode of metabolism of T_3s (rT_3 and T_3). Two T_2s, 3,3'-T_2 and 3',5'-T_2, could derive from the metabolism of 3,3',5'-T_3 (rT_3) (Fig. 8.1). Both of these have been demonstrated in human circulation. Serum levels of 3,3'-T_2 as well as 3',5'-T_2 increase considerably after oral administration of rT_3 (Wu et al. 1976; Chopra et al. 1978 d; Geola et al. 1979). Similarly, radioactive 3,3'-T_2 and 3',5'-T_2 have been found in human plasma after intravenous administration of rT_3 labeled in the phenolic (outer) ring. Studies of thyroid glands hydrolyzed with pronase suggest that the 3,3'-T_2 and 3',5'-T_2 content of human thyroglobulin is very low on a weight basis, approximating only about 0.05% and 0.06% that of T_4, respectively.

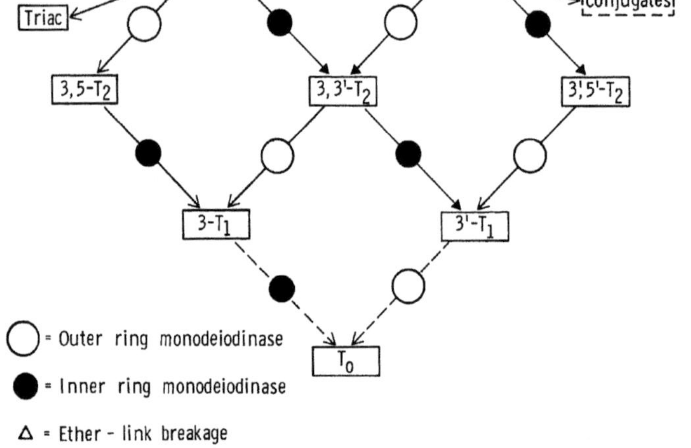

Fig. 8.1. A schematic view of a possible cascade of metabolism of T_4 and its deiodinated derivatives. *Dotted lines* mark those areas where data on the operation of a pathway or the existence of a compound are either not available or insufficient. * = DIT could also be produced by breakage of ether linkage of 3,5-T_2. ** = MIT could also be produced by breakage of ether linkage of 3.3'-T_2 and 3-T_1

Assuming that T_4 and the T_2s are secreted in the same proportion as is present in the thyroglobulin and knowing the MCRs of 3,3'-T_2 (~560 liters/day) and 3',5'-T_2 (~159 liters/day) and T_4 (~1.18 liters/day), it can be calculated that the thyroidal secretion that results in a normal serum T_4 concentration of 7.5 µg/dl, contributes less than 1% to serum concentration of 3,3'-T_2 (~4 ng/dl) or 3',5'-T_2 (~6 ng/100 ml) in normal man (Chopra et al. 1978 d; Geola et al. 1979). These analyses suggest that the bulk of 3,3'-T_2 and 3',5'-T_2 in the human circulation derive from the peripheral metabolism of T_3s.

As in the case of rT_3, the metabolism of 3,5,3'-T_3 can also lead to two T_2s: 3,3'-T_2 and 3,5-T_2. The serum concentration of 3,3'-T_2 increases after oral administration of T_3 (Wu et al. 1976; Gavin et al. 1978), and radioactive 3,3'-T_2 has been demonstrated in human plasma after intravenous administration T_3 labeled in the phenolic ring (Rudolph et al. 1978); 3,5-T_2 has also been demonstrated in human serum by RIA. Reported mean serum values vary considerably between <1 and 7 ng/100 ml (Meinhold and Schurnabrand 1978; Maciel et al. 1979 b: Pangaro et al. 1979; Engler et al. 1979). A study of the conversion of T_3 to 3,5-T_2 in vivo has been difficult because of contamination of commercial T_3 with 3,5-T_2. However, the thyroidal content of 3,5-T_2 is only about 0.07% that of T_4, which suggests that, as in the case of other T_2s, thyroidal secretion probably contributes very minimally to 3,5-T_2 in the serum of normal man, and that the bulk of this T_2 in human serum probably derives from peripheral metabolism of T_3 (Pangaro et al. 1979; Maciel et al. 1979 b).

Gavin et al. (1978) examined the daily PRs of one of the two deiodinative metabolites of T_3, i. e., 3,3'-T_2, in three hypothyroid patients treated with T_3 (40–80 µg/day). In these patients PR-3,3'-T_2 ranged between 29% and 75% of PR-T_3. The daily PR of the other T_2 that may be produced from the metabolism of T_3 is not known at this time. Geola et al. (1979) examined the daily PRs of 3',5'-T_2 and rT_3 in normal subjects; the ratio of PR-3',5'-T_2 and PR-rT_3 (3',5'-T_2/rT_3) ranged between 18% and 62%, suggesting that 38%–82% of rT_3 produced daily may be metabolized by conversion to 3,3'-T_2 and/or via other nondeiodinative routes of metabolism. More detailed and simultaneous study of PRs of T_3s, as well as all three possible T_2s (3,3'-T_2, 3',5'-T_2, and 3,5-T_2), are required to attain a complete understanding of the various deiodinative routes of metabolism of T_3s.

In addition to deiodination, T_3s may be metabolized by conjugation to glucuronide and the sulfate forms, and by conversion to acetic acid analogues (triiodothyroacetic acid, TRIAC, in the case of T_3, and reverse-TRIAC, in the case of rT_3). There is no information available on the serum concentrations of the conjugates of T_3 or rT_3. TRIAC has been demonstrated in human serum with a mean normal concentration approximating 2–5 ng/dl (Nakamura et al. 1978; Livermore et al. 1979). The conversion of D-T_3 to D-TRIAC has been shown in vivo in man (Burger A, cited in Chopra et al. 1978c), but it is not known how much of normal serum TRIAC concentration derives from the metabolism of T_3 and how much from the outer-ring monodeiodination of TETRAC. Recent studies show, however, that some 10% of T_3 produced in euthyroid individuals may be metabolized by conversion to TRIAC (Livermore et al. 1979). Reverse TRIAC has not yet been quantified in human serum. Simultaneous information on the production rates of T_3 and rT_3, their conjugates, and TRIAC and reverse TRIAC is required to assess the relative quantitative significance of nondeiodinative routes of metabolism of T_3s.

Some T_3 is also lost in the urine as T_3, but the urinary excretion of T_3 (~0.6 μg/day. Rogowski et al. 1978) normally constitutes only about 2% of daily PR-T_3. The amount of rT_3 excreted in the urine of a euthyroid individual, about 72 ng/day (Faber et al. 1978), is very low (~0.2% of PR-rT_3), apparently because it is deiodinated to T_2s even more rapidly than is T_3. Urinary excretion of rT_3 is increased to about 184 ng/day in hyperthyroidism, whereas it is decreased to about 29 ng/day in hypothyroidism (Faber et al. 1978).

B. In Vitro Studies

The processes of outer-ring monodeiodination of rT_3 and of inner-ring monodeiodination of T_3 to 3,3′-T_2 have been examined in vitro using rat tissue homogenates (Chopra et al. 1978 a; Visser et al. 1978 b). 3,3′-T_2 was produced regularly when either substrate (rT_3 and T_3) was incubated with homogenates of liver or kidney; other tissues generated little or no T_2. More detailed studies with liver homogenate suggest that rT_3 to 3,3′-T_2 as well as T_3 to 3′3-T_2 generating activities are influenced significantly by substrate concentration, tissue concentration, pH, temperature, and duration of incubation. The important influences of substrate concentration, pH, and temperature suggest that both activities are enzymic in nature. The apparent Km for rT_3 to 3,3′-T_2 conversion approximates 65 n*M*, while that for T_3 to T_2 conversion is about 6 μ*M*. T_2 production is maximal or near maximal from both substrates at a pH between 7.8 and 8.5 and at 37° C. Since 3,3′-T_2 is degraded very rapidly at pH 6.5, the optimal pH ranges noted above may have to be modified when purified preparations of the monodeiodinases become available.

Both rT_3 and T_3 to 3,3′-T_2 converting activities are unaffected by large doses of sodium iodide, diiodotyrosine (DIT), and methimazole. They are inhibited in a dose-dependent manner by propylthiouracil, iodoacetic acid, ipodate, and dinitrophenol. Propylthiouracil and iodoacetic acid inhibit T_2 production from rT_3 as well as T_3 in an uncompetitive and noncompetitive manner, respectively. Both reactions are stimulated by thiol agents (e. g., dithiothreitol and reduced glutathione). Reverse T_3 to 3, 3′-T_2 converting activity is inhibited by an SH oxidizing agent, diamide, as well as by SH binding reagents, *N*-ethylmaleimide and mercuric chloride (Chopra et al. 1978 a; Chopra 1978 b). Similar studies of the effects of SH-oxidizing or reducing agents have not been well documented in the case of T_3 to 3,3′-T_2 converting activity.

The similarities of characteristics, as well as organ distribution of activities monodeiodinating T_4, T_3, and rT_3, raise a question of whether these are the same or similar activities. The question is a particularly important one in the case of enzymes that monodeiodinate T_4 and rT_3 in the outer ring to T_3 and 3,3′-T_2, respectively. These activities not only have similar organ distribution, similar dependence on SH groups, and similar inhibition by propylthiouracil, iodoacetic acid, and sodium ipodate, but they also have a similar subcellular location in the plasma membranes. Furthermore, rT_3 inhibits the conversion of T_4 to T_3 in a competitive manner, and T_4 inhibits conversion of rT_3 to 3,3′-T_2, presumably in a competitive manner as well (Chopra 1977; Kaplan and Utiger 1978 a). The only major difference between the converting activities of T_4 to T_3 and of rT_3 to 3,3′T_2 is in the Km for the substrate; the Km for rT_3 to T_2 monodeiodination is some 40- to 100-fold lower than that for

T_4 to T_3 monodeiodination (~2.5 μ*M*). If the monodeiodinases acting on T_4 and rT_3 are the same, then it may seem that monodeiodinase was devised teleologically for the degradation of rT_3, and that the "fit" or reaction of T_4 is a matter of cross-reaction. This may seem to be a rather casual and fortuitous arrangement for so important a biologic reaction as the conversion of T_4 to T_3. In any case, similarity between T_4 and rT_3 outer-ring monodeiodinating activities is a confounding one. It actually makes one wonder whether there is just one outer-ring monodeiodinase for the metabolism of iodothyronines or a family of closely related outer-ring (and a separate set of inner-ring) monodeiodinases. The question would be answered satisfactorily if methods for isolation of iodothyronine monodeiodinases were to become available.

There is no information at present about the nature of or the factors influencing the monodeiodination of rT_3 to 3′,5′-T_2 and monodeiodination of T_3 to 3,5-T_2. Similarly no new data are available on factors that influence nondeiodinative modes of metabolism of T_3 (or rT_3) to TRIAC (or reverse TRIAC) (see Tomita et al. 1957; Galton and Pitt-Rivers 1959 for a review of existing information) or to T_3 (or rT_3) conjugates.

In vitro studies have also demonstrated the production of iodotyrosines (DIT) when T_4 was incubated with tissue homogenate (Plaskett 1961; Wynn and Gibbs 1962; Roche et al. 1962). A recent study confirmed this pathway of metabolism of T_4 (Balsam and Ingbar 1979). However, the quantitative significance of the metabolic pathway remains uncertain. The consensus of the opinion at this time seems to be that sequential monodeiodination, and not breakage of ether linkage, is the predominant mode of metabolism of iodothyronines and that thyronine is the ultimate degradative product of the metabolism. Demonstration by Pittman and Chambers (1969) of intact thyronine in urine of rats given carbon-labeled T_4 favors the concept of sequential stripping of iodine atoms as the main mechanism in the metabolism of iodothyronines.

Chapter 9

Biologic Effects of Iodothyronines

The biologic effects of thyroid hormones vary with different species (e.g., metamorphosis in the tadpole), as well as with the stage of development within a species (fetal vs. adult life). Table 9.1 lists some effects of thyroid hormones on various systems, some of which are interdependent. Thus, the influence of thyroid hormones on cellular differentiation, growth, and development in the fetal and neonatal period apparently reflects gene expression manisfested via increased synthesis of new proteins and enzymes, and/or by activation of the existing enzymes. Similarly, thyroid hormones induce stimulation of oxygen consumption in the tissues which appears importantly related (but not entirely) to new synthesis as well as activation of ouabain-sensitive Na^+ K^+ ATPase in the cell membrane (Lo and

Table 9.1. Some biological effects of thyroid hormone[a]

I	Cellular differentiation and growth, especially in the fetal and neonatal period, e.g., tadpole metamorphosis, cerebral cortical and cerebellar growth, myelination, and differentiation	
II	Stimulation of oxygen consumption by the tissues, e.g., liver, kidney, muscle. Spleen, testes, and adult brain respond poorly to this effect of thyroid hormones	
III	Suppression of pituitary TSH synthesis and release[b]	
IV	Retardation of amino acid efflux from the cells	
V	Regulation of synthesis of proteins and enzymes, e.g.	
	Increased synthesis:	Skin epidermis and hair
		hypophyseal hormones: growth hormone, prolactin
		Cell membrane Na, K-ATPase
		mitochondrial—glycerophosphate dehydrogenase
		glycolytic enzymes including NAD-specific isocitric dehydrogenase, hexokinase, malic enzyme, glucose 6-phosphate dehydrogenase, etc.
	Decreased synthesis, e.g., mitochondrial NADP-linked isocitric dehydrogenase in rats given thyroid hormones	
VI	Activation of enzymes, e.g.	
	Na, K-ATPase	
	Cytochromes	
	Disphosphoglycerate mutase that results in formation of 2,3-diphosphoglycerate in erythrocytes	
	L-T_3 aminotransferase in the liver	
VII	Conversion of carotenes to vitamin A	
VIII	Stimulation of erythropoietin mediated erythropoeisis	
IX	Inhibition of phosphodiesterase in the cartilage	
X	Interaction with other hormones e.g., stimulation (or inhibition in case of rT_3) of lipolytic action of epinephrine, ACTH, and glucagon	

[a] Adapted in part from Shambaugh (1978)

[b] Effects I–III may be related to IV–VI.

Edelman 1976). Evidence exists to suggest that TSH suppressive effects of thyroid hormones may also be mediated via synthesis of a protein (Bowers et al. 1968).

A. Mechanism of Action

A currently popular model for the effects of thyorid hormones envisages the following sequence of events: (1) entry of free hormone into the cell via penetration of the cell membrane, (2) binding by one or more of the cytosolic proteins, (3) existence of an equilibrium between cytosol bound and unbound thyroid hormone, (4) uptake of free hormone by specific high-affinity, low-capacity binding sites in acidic nonhistone receptor proteins in the nuclear chromatin, (5) increased transcriptional activity and increased formation and release into cytosol of messenger ribonucleic acid (mRNA), and (6) increased translational activity and increased synthesis of proteins and enzymes (Oppenheimer et al. 1976). Studies of Tata (1969) have played an important role in the generation of this scheme. Following a single injection of T_3 into a thyroidectomized rat, Tata recorded in liver an increased synthesis of nuclear RNA at 5–10 h, increased DNA-dependent RNA polymerase activity in nuclei at 12–15 h, a clear increase in ribosomal RNA at about 24 h, increased synthesis of proteins from amino acids at about 35–40 h, followed soon thereafter by increased oxygen consumption. An increase in liver size was evident at about 70 h.

Certain studies suggest that binding to nuclear chromatin and the resulting changes in protein synthesis may not be the only way that thyroid hormones exert their effects. Sterling et al. (1977) obtained good evidence for the existence of high-affinity binding sites for thyroid hormones in the inner membrane layer of the mitochondria. They believe that the binding of thyroid hormones to mitochondria may be at least as important as (and possibly even more important than) the binding to the nuclei in stimulation of the oxygen consumption by the thyroid hormones (Sterling et al. 1977; Sterling 1979).

Direct effects of the thyroid hormones on the cell membranes have also been well documented. Adamson and Ingbar (1967) showed an increased incorporation of neutral amino acids into embryonic chick bone and rat cartilage in vitro which was not inhibited by the presence in the incubation medium of puromycin or actinomycin D. Goldfine et al. (1976) reported an increased uptake of cycloleucine and aminoisobutyrate by rat thymocytes in the presence of T_3 or T_4. This effect of T_3, which resulted from a reduced efflux of amino acids from the thymocyte, was not inhibited by a reduction in protein synthesis by cyclcheximide. However, high concentrations of T_3 (or T_4), about 10^{-7}–$10^{-6}M$, were required to detect the responses mentioned above. More recently, Blanchard and Davis (1978) have shown activation of Na^+-K^+ ATPase in renal cortical cells in vitro with as low a concentration as $10^{-15}M$ of T_3. This effect too was not blocked by cycloheximide, an inhibitor of protein synthesis. Overall, it seems then that thyroid hormones may influence tissues by a combination of their effects on the nuclei, the mitochondria, and the plasma membranes.

B. Some Other Interesting Effects of Thyroid Hormones

I. Erythropoiesis

Several recent studies have focused on the effects of thyroid hormones in addition to calorigenesis and TSH suppression. The studies of thyroid hormone effects on erythropoiesis are especially interesting. These studies show that thyroid hormones influence the production of erythropoietin as well as its effect in vitro on differentiation and growth of hematopoietic precursors. Studies of canine and human erythroid cells showed that this effect may be mediated by surface receptors with β_2 subspecificity. A β-adrenergic inhibitor, propranolol, is a potent inhibitor of the effects of thyroid hormones on the erythroid precursors (Golde et al. 1977; Popovic et al. 1977; Dianik et al. 1978).

II. Cyclic (3′,5′-) Adenosine Monophosphate

Thyroid hormones also influence the metabolism of cyclic 3′,5′-adenosine monophosphate (AMP). They have been shown to stimulate the synthesis of AMP in cardiac muscle and to inhibit AMP phosphodiesterase in adipose tissue, frog erythrocytes, and rat calvaria (Levey and Epstein 1969; Mandel und Kuehl 1967; Solomon 1972; Marcus 1975). The T_3-induced reduction in phosphodiesterase and resulting increase in AMP content of adipose tissue may be responsible for the increase in lipolysis following treatment with thyroid hormones (Mandel and Kuehl 1967). Whether or not a similar mechanism is involved in the increased rate of bone turnover in hyperthyroidism is not clear. The concentrations of T_4 (or T_3) that inhibited phosphodiesterase in rat calvaria were very high ($\sim 10^{-5}$ *M*) (Marcus 1975). It is not known whether the requirement of high doses was a function of a general insensitivity of in vitro preparation, inordinate nonspecific binding by tissue proteins, or a combination of these factors, or if the effect of thyroid hormones on phosphodiesterase is not a physiologic one.

III. Self Degradation

Recent studies also suggest a possibility that thyroid hormones influence their own degradation via transamination to pyruvic acid metabolites. The administration of T_3 (or T_4) to normal and hypothyroid rats increases the activity of L-T_3 aminotransferase. Interestingly, rT_3 was found to be as active as T_3 in enhancing hepatic L-T_3 aminotransferase activity (Fishman et al. 1977). However, although the product of transamination of T_3, i.e., triiodothyropyruvic acid, has been demonstrated in rat liver after T_3 administration (Michel et al. 1962), the overall significance of transamination in the metabolism of T_3 is uncertain at this time.

C. Relative Potency in Various Effects

Table 9.2 presents data on the relative potencies of various iodothyronines and their analogue associated with various biologic effects. It is clear that T_3 is the most

Table 9.2. Comparison of biologic effects of naturally occurring iodothyronines with T_4 set at 100

Assay System	Function tested[a]	References	T_3	rT_3	$3,3'T_2$	$3'5'T_2$	$3,5T_2$	$3'T_1$	To	TETRAC	TRIAC
Tadpole metamorphosis	I	Money et al. 1960; Cortell, 1949	300–1000	2–5[b]	25–70[b]	–	0–40[b]	0[b]	0	200–1300	2400–12000
Stimulation of BMR	II	Money et al. 1960; Tomich et al. 1960; Gaddum 1930	200–800	<1	<3	<1[b]	11[b]	<1		11	21
Goiter prevention assay	III	Money et al. 1960; Cortell 1949; Tomich et al. 1960	300–1000	<3	<1–100[b]	<3	9	<1[b]	0	57–100	51–100
Thyroidal radioiodine suppression	III	Money et al. 1960; Cortell 1949; Tomich et al. 1960	300–500	<1–10[b]	70–100[b]		37[b]			75	75

[a] Numbers here correspond to numbers in Table 9.1.
[b] DL isomer was studied for this effect.

Continued next page

Table 9.2 (continued)

Assay System	Function tested[a]	References	T_3	rT_3	$3,3'T_2$	$3'5'T_2$	$3,5T_2$	$3'T_1$	To	TETRAC	TRIAC
In vitro reduction of TSH response to TRH	III	Chopra et al. 1978b	800–1600	8–11	~8	–	–			–	–
Binding to nuclear proteins	III	Rat liver: Koerner et al. 1974, 1975;	1000	1	–	–	–			150	1640
		Latham et al. 1976.	500	25	–	–	–	–		–	–
		Human lymphocytes: Lemarchand-Beraud et al. 1978	200	100	–	–	–	–		–	200
Amino acid transport to embryonic chick bone	IV	Adamson and Ingbar 1967	100–200	50–100[b]	100[b]	–	~50	–	0	–	–
Amino acid transport in rat thymocytes	IV	Goldfine et al. 1975, 1976	300	140	300	15[b]	44	9	0	–	–
Activation of L-T_3 amino transferase in rat liver	V or VI	Fishman et al. 1977	100	100	–	–	–	–	–	–	–

Stimulation of Na, K ATPase in isolated kidney cells in vitro	VI	Blanchard and Davis 1978, 1979	100	–	–	–	–	–	–	< 1	–
Stimulation of erythro-poiesis	VIII	Golde et al. 1977; Dianik et al. 1978	100–1000	~100	–	–	–	–	–	~200	~200
Inhibition of phospho-diesterase in rat adipocytes	IX	Marcus 1975; Marcus et al. 1975	27	25–50	25	–	<10	–	0	1720	248
Influence on epinephrine induced lipo-lysis in rat adipocytes	X	Hagg et al. 1978	stimula-tory	in-hibi-tory	–	–	–	–	–	–	–

potent agent in most effects including augmentation of oxygen consumption and inhibition of TSH secretion. T_4 is the next most potent agent; observation of significant in vivo conversation of T_4 to T_3 has suggested that at least some, and possibly a large fraction, of the effect of T_4 is attributable to its conversion to T_3. Some in vitro studies do make a case, however, that T_4 is able to affect the suppression of TSH from the pituitary under conditions in which little or no conversion to T_3 is demonstrable (Chopra et al. 1978 b). This finding leads one to consider that, although conversion to T_3 is an efficient mode of action of T_4, it may not be absolutely necessary. The finding of normal serum TSH and essentially a normal TSH response to TRH in several instances of low-T_3 syndrome (see Chap. 4) supports this consideration.

Examination of Table 9.2 highlights another interesting aspect of the biologic effects of iodothyronines. It shows that rT_3, 3,3′-T_2, and 3,5-T_2, which have little or no ability to stimulate oxygen consumption or suppression of TSH secretion, are quite active with respect to some other biologic effects. Thus, T_3 is comparable to T_4, while 3,3′-T_2 is even more active than T_4, in increasing amino acid transport in chick bone and thymocytes. Similarly, rT_3 is nearly as active as T_3 in increasing erythropoietin-stimulated proliferation and differentiation of erythroid precursors, in inhibiting phosphodiesterase and activating hepatic L-T_3 aminotransferase. Curiously, rT_3 works in a direction opposite to that of T_3 in some other biologic systems. Thus, whereas treatment with T_3 increases oxygen consumption, administration of rT_3 in pharmacologic doses to hyperthyroid patients has been found associated with a reduction in the BMR (Benua et al. 1959). Reverse T_3 is also a potent inhibitor of the conversion of T_4 to T_3 by homogenates of rat liver or kidney in vitro, while treatment of rats with T_3 (or T_4) enhances the ability of their tissues to generate T_3 from T_4 (Kaplan and Utiger 1978). Hagg et al. (1978) have recently shown that, whereas T_3 enhances the epinephrine-mediated increase in lipolysis from rat adipocytes, rT_3 has a dose-dependent inhibitory effect. Reverse T_3 was also observed to overcome the enhancement of epinephrine-stimulated lipolysis produced by up to a 10-fold higher dose of T_3. Unliker rT_3 (and like T_3), 3,5-T_2 is a potent stimulator of lypolysis in adipose tissue (Mandel and Kuehl 1967).

The doses of iodothyronines used in most in vitro studies of thyroid hormone effects other than calorigenesis and TSH suppression have, in general, tended to be supraphysiologic. Therefore, it is not clear whether or not the effects observed are directly pertinent to physiologic circumstances. However, the available data do clearly make a case that the iodothyronines present in biologic fluids in addition to T_3 and T_4 are not merely inert degradative metabolites of thyroid hormones and that they are capable of some biologic effects. The high doses required to show some effect in vitro may reflect the artificiality of in vitro sytems used or they may suggest than an appropriate effect has not been studied. It seems quite possible that various normally occurring metabolites of T_4 and T_3, as well as their analogues are intended for specialized effects of iodothyronines distinct from calorigenesis or TSH suppression, which may be as important as, or under some circumstances even more important than, calorigenesis or TSH suppression. The effects of these metabolites may become manifest at the site of their origin or in the organs involved in their removal from the circulation. It is hoped that further work along this line of inquiry will bring forth interesting information on thyroid hormone physiology in health or disease.

References

Abrams GM, Larsen PR (1973) Triiodothyronine and thyroxine in the serum and thyroid glands of iodine deficient rats. J Clin Invest 52:2522

Abuid JL, Klein AH, Foley TP jr, Larsen PR (1974) Total and free triiodothyronine and thyroxine in early infancy. J. Clin Endocrinol Metab 39:263

Adamson LF, Ingbar SH (1967) Selective alteration by triiodothyronine of amino acid transport in embryonic bone. Endocrinology 81:1362

Aickin CM, Fraser S, Cooper E, Hall G, Burke CW (1977) Thyroid hormone kinetics: improved method for quantitative separation and measurement of the various radioiodinated species in serum after radioiodothyronine injection. Clin Endocrinol (Oxf) 7:469

Albright EC, Larson FC (1959) Metabolism of L-thyroxine by human tissue slices. J Clin Invest 38:1899

Albright EC, Larson FC, Tust RH (1954) In vitro conversion of thyroxine to triiodothyronine by kidney slices. Proc Soc Exp Biol Med 86:137

Andrea TA (1977) Thyroid hormone analogs: Synthesis, antigoitre activities, decomposition of the thermodynamic functions of binding, conformational population analysis and binding to prealbumin. PhD thesis, University of California

Andrea TA, Dietrich SW, Murray WJ, Kollman PA, Jorgensen EC (1979) A model for thyroid hormone receptor interactions. J Med Chem 22:221

Andrea TA, Jorgensen EC, Kollman PA (1978) Differentiation of D- and L-thyroxine by the plasma protein prealbumin. Int J Quantum Chem 5, 191

Aron M, van Caulaert C, Stahl J (1931) L'equilibre entre l'hormone prehypophysaire et l'hormone thyroidienne dans le milieu interier a l'état normal et a l'état pathologigue. C R Soc Biol (Paris) 107:64

Av Ruskin TW, Tang SC, Shenkman G, Mitsuma T, Hollander CS (1973) Serum triiodothyronine concentrations in infancy, childhood and adolescence and pediatric thyroid disorders. J Clin Endocrinol Metab 37:235

Balfour WE, Tunnicliffe HE (1960) Thyroxine binding by serum proteins. J. Physiol (Lond) 53:179

Balsam A, Ingbar SH (1978a) The influence of fasting, diabetes and several pharmacological agents on the pathways of thyroxine metabolism in rat liver. J Clin Invest 62:415

Balsam A, Ingbar SH (1978 b) The mechanism of regulation of triiodothyronine (T_3) generation from thyroxine (T_4) in liver of normal and fasted rats. Clin Res 26:489A

Balsam A, Ingbar SH (1979) Ether-link cleavage: an alternate pathway of thyroxine metabolism. Clin Res 27:247A

Balsam A, Sexton F, Ingbar SH (1977) Independent inhibitory effects of hypothyroidism and fasting on hepatic conversion of thyroxine (T_4) to triiodothyronine (T_3) in the rat. Annu Meet Endocr Soc, abstract 365

Barker SB, Pittman CS, Pittman JA jr, Hill SR jr (1960) Thyroxine antagonism by partially iodinated thyronines and analogues. Ann NY Acad Sci 86:545

Basedow CA von (1840) Exophthalmos durch Hypertrophie des Zellgewebes in der Augenhöhle. Wochenschr Heilkd 6:197, 220

Baumann E (1896) Über das Thyrojodin. MMW 43:309

Baur WH (1972) Prediction of hydrogen bonds and hydrogen atom positions in crystalline solids. Acta Cryst allogr B28:1456

Becker RA, Johnson DW, Wilmore DW, Burman KD, Wartofsky L, Woeber KA (1976) Alterations in serum triiodothyronine and reverse triiodothyronine in thermal injury. Clin Res 24:269A

Bellabarba D, Inada D, Versano — Abaron N, Sterling K (1968) Thyroxine transport and turnover in major nonthyroidal illness. J Clin Endocrinol Metab 28:1023

Bennoti JR, Grimaldi R, Pino S, Maloof F (1970) A modified method for total triiodothyronine (T_3) by competitive protein binding. 6th Internat Thyroid Conf, Vienna, Austria, P. 139, abstract 127
Benua RS, Kumaoka S, Leeper RD, Rawson RW (1959) The effect of dl-3,3',5'-triiodothyronine in Graves' disease. J Clin Endocrinol Metab 19:1344
Bermudez F, Surks MI, Oppenheimer JH (1975) High incidence of decreased serum triiodothyronine concentration in patients with nonthyroidal disease. J Clin Endocrinol Metab 41:27
Berson SA, Yalow RS (1954) Quantitative aspects of iodine metabolism. The exchangeable organic iodine pool, and the rates of thyroidal secretion, peripheral degradation and fecal excretion of endogenously synthesized organically bound iodine. J Clin Invest 33:1533
Bianchi R, Zucchelli GC, Giannessi D, Pilo A, Mariani C, Carpi A, Toni MG, Cazzuola F (1978) Evaluation of triiodothyronine (T_3) kinetics in normal subjects, in hypothyroid, and hyperthyroid patients using specific anti-serum for the determination of labeled T_3 in plasma. J Clin Endocrinol Metab 46:203
Birkhauser M, Busset R, Burer R Burger A (1977) Diagnosis of hyperthyroidism when serum thyroxine alone is raised. Lancet II:53
Blake CCF, Oatley SJ (1977) Protein-DNA and protein-hormone interactions in prealbumin: a model of the thyroid hormone nuclear receptor? Nature 268:115
Blake CCF, Geisow MJ, Swan IDA, Rerat C, Rerat B (1974) Structure of human plasma prealbumin at 2.5A resolution. J Mol Biol 88:1
Blanchard RF, Davis PJ (1978) Dependence of renal Na, K-adenosine triphosphatase on subphysiologic levels of thyroid hormone in vitro. Ann Meet Amer Thyroid Assoc, pp T–19
Blanchard RF, Davis PJ (1979) Specific interaction of thyroid hormones with rat renal Na, K-ATPase in vitro: evidence for non-nuclear activation of enzyme. Clin Res 27:248A
Bolger MB (1978) Molecular interactions between thyroid hormone analogs and the solubilized rat liver nuclear receptor. PhD dissertation, University of California
Bondi A (1964) Van der Waals volumes and radii. J Phys Chem 68:441
Bowers CY, Lee KL, Schally AU (1968) A study on the interaction of the thyrotropin-releasing factor and L-triiodothyronine: effects of puromycin and cycloheximide. Endocrinology 82:75
Branch WT jr, Pages RA, Cahnmann HJ, Edelhoch H, Robbins J (1971) Thyroxine binding prealbumin as a model for thyroxine – protein interactions. Annu Meet Amer. Thyroid Assoc, p 65
Brandt N, Kehlet H, Hansen JM, Skovsted L (1976) Serum triiodothyronine and surgery. Lancet I:491
Braverman LE, Socolow EL, Woeber KA, Ingbar SH (1968) Effect of norethandrolone on the metabolism of ^{125}I-labeled thyroxine binding prealbumin. J Clin Endocrinol Metab 28:831
Braverman LE, Ingbar SH, Sterling K (1970) Conversion of thyroxine (T_4) to triiodothyronine (T_3) in athyrotic human subjects. J Clin Invest 49:855
Brooks MH, Waldstein SS, Bronsky D, Sterling K (1975) Serum triiodothyronine concentration in thyroid storm. J Clin Endocrinol Metab 40:339
Brown BL, Ekins RP, Ellis SM, Reith WS (1970) Specific antibodies to triiodothyronine hormone. Nature 226:359
Brown BL, Ekins RP, Ellis SM, Reith WS (1971) The radioimmunoassay of triiodothyronine. In: Further advances in thyroid research, vol 2. K Fellinger, R Hofer (eds), Verlag der Wiener Medizinischen Akademie, Vienna, Vol 2, p 1107
Brown J, Solomon DH, Beall GN, Terasaki PI, Chopra IJ, van Herle AJ, Wu SY (1978) Autoimmune thyroid diseases – Graves' and Hashimoto's. Ann Intern Med 88:379
Brunell P, Bohuon C (1972) Baisse de la triiodothyronine serique avec l'age. Clin Chim Acta 42:201
Burger A, Ingbar SH (1974) Labeling of thyroid hormones and their derivatives. Endocrinology 94:1189
Burger A, Sakoloff C. (1977) Serum 3,3'-L-diiodothyronine, a direct radioimmunoassay in human serum: method and clinical results. J Clin Endocrinol Metab 45:384
Burger A. Sakoloff C, Staeheli V, Valloton MB, Ingbar SH (1975) Radioimmunoassays of 3,5,3'-triiodo-L-thyronine with and without a prior extraction step. Acta Endocrinol (Copenh) 80:58
Burger A, Dinichert D, Nicod P, Jenny M, Lemarchand-Beraud T, Vallotton MB (1976 a) Effect of amiodarone on serum triiodothyronine, reverse triiodothyronine, thyroxine and thyrotropin: a drug influencing peripheral metabolism of thyroid hormones. J Clin Invest 58:255
Burger A, Suter P, Nicod P, Vallotton MB, Vagenakis A, Braverman L (1976 b) Reduced active thyroid hormone levels in acute illness. Lancet I:653
Burger AG, Wimpfheimer C, Burger A, Danforth E jr (1978) Lack of relationship between starvation ketosis and serum T_3 levels. Annu Meet Endocr Soc, p 115 abstract 81

Burgi H, Wimpfheimer C, Burger A, Zaunbauer W, Rosler H, Lemarchand-Beraud T (1976) Changes of circulating thyroxine, triiodothyronine, and reverse triiodothyronine after radiographic contrast agents. J Clin Endocrinol Metab 43:1203

Burgus R, Dunn TF, Ward DN, Vale W, Amoss M, Guillemin R (1969) Dérives polypeptidiques de synthèsedoues d'active hypophysiotrope TRF. C R Acad Sci [D] (Paris) 268, 2116 (1969)

Burman KD, Strum D, Dimonond RC, Djuh YY, Wright FD, Earll JD, Wartofsky L (1977 a) A radioimmunoassay for 3,3'-L-diiodothyronine (3,3'-T_2). J Clin Endocrinol Metab 45:339

Burman KD, Dimond RC, Wright FD, Earll JM, Bruton J, Wartofsky L (1977 b) A radioimmunoassay for 3,3',5'-L-triiodothyronine (reverse T_3): assessment of thyroid gland content and serum measurements in conditions of normal and altered thyroidal economy and following administration of thyrotropin releasing hormone (TRH) and thyrotropin (TSH). J Clin Endocrinol Metab 44:660

Burr WA, Black EG, Griffiths RS, Hoffenberg R, Meinhold H, Wenzel KW (1975) Serum triiodothyronine and reverse triiodothyronine concentrations after surgical operation. Lancet II: 1277

Burr WA, Griffiths RS, Ramsden DB, Black EG, Hoffenberg R (1976) Effect of a single dose of dexamethasone on serum concentrations of thyroid hormones. Lancet II: 58

Burrows AW, Cooper E, Shakespeare RA, Aickin CM, Fraser S, Hesch RD, Burke CW (1977) Low serum L-T_3 levels in the elderly sick: protein binding, thyroid and pituitary responsiveness and reverse T_3 concentrations. Clin Endocrinol 7:289

Burse RL, Goldman RF, Danforth E, Robbin DC, Horton ES, Sim EAH (1977) Effect of excess protein on metabolism. Physiologist 20:13

Camerman A, Camerman N (1974 a) Thyroid hormone stereochemistry. I. The molecular structure of 3,5,3'-triiodo-L-thyronine (T_3) and L-thyroxine (T_4). Acta Crystallogr B30:1832

Camerman A, Camerman N (1974 b) Thyroid hormone stereochemistry. II. Molecular structure of thyronine. HCl ethyl ester monohydrate. Can J Chem 52:3042

Camerman N, Camerman A (1974) Thyroid hormone stereochemistry. III. Molecular structure of triiodothyropropionic acid ethyl ester. Can J Chem 52:3048

Camerman N, Fawcett JK, Reynolds WF, Camerman A (1975) Thyroid hormone conformation from NMR studies of triiodothyropropionic acid. Nature 253:50

Carlson HE, Drenick EJ, Chopra IJ, Hershman JM (1977) Alterations in basal and TRH-stimulated serum levels of thyrotrophin, prolactin, and thyroid hormones in starved obese men. J Clin Endocrinol Metab 45:707

Carter JN, Eastman CJ, Corcoran JM, Lazarus L (1974) Effect of severe chronic illness on thyroid function. Lancet II:971

Cavalieri RR, Searle GL, Castle JN, Dickard R (1966) The kinetics of ^{131}I-labeled L-thyroxine in man: observations of subjects with normal and decreased serum thyroxine binding globulin. J Clin Invest 45:939

Cavalieri RR, Steinberg M, Searle GL (1970). The distribution kinetics of triiodothyronine: studies of euthyroid subjects with decreased plasma thyroxine binding globulin and patients with Graves' disease. J Clin Invest 49:1041

Cavalieri RR, Steinberg M, Searle GL (1971) Metabolic clearance rate of L-triiodothyronine in man: a comparison of results by single injection and constant infusion methods. J Clin Endocrinol Metab 33:624

Cavalieri RR, McMohan FA, Castle JN (1975) Preparation of ^{125}I-labeled human thyroxine binding alpha globulin and its turnover in normal and hypothyroid subjects. J. Clin Invest 56:79

Cavalieri RR, Gavin LA, Bui F (1977) Conversion of thyroxine to 3,3',5'-triiodothyronine (reverse T_3) by a soluble enzyme system of rat liver. Biochem Biophys Res Commun 79:897

Chan V, Landon J, Besser GM, Ekins RP (1972) Urinary triiodothyronine excretion as index of thyroid function. Lancet II:253

Cheng SY, Cahnmann HJ, Wilchek M, Ferguson RN (1975) Affinity labeling of the thyroxine binding domain of human serum prealbumin with dansyl chloride. Biochemistry 14:4132

Cheng SY, Wilchek M, Cahnman HJ, Robbins J (1977) Affinity labeling of human serum prealbumin with N-bromo-acetyl-L-thyroxine. J Biol Chem 252:6076

Chiraseveenprapund P, Buergi U, Goswami A, Rosenberg IN (1976) Conversion of L-thyroxine to triiodothyronine in rat kidney homogenate, in thyroid research. Excerpta Medica, Amsterdam, p 239

Chiraseveenprapund P, Buergi U, Goswami A, Rosenberg IN (1978) Conversion of L-thyroxine to triiodothyronine in rat kidney homogenate. Endocrinology 102:12

Chopra IJ (1971) An improved radioimmunoassay (RIA) for measurement of thyroxine (T_4) in serum. Annu Meet Amer Thyroid Assoc, p 453

Chopra IJ (1972) A radioimmunoassay of thyroxine in unextracted serum. J Clin Endocrinol Metab 34:938

Chopra IJ (1974) A radioimmunoassay for measurement of 3,3′,5′-triiodothyronine (reverse T_3). J Clin Invest 54:583

Chopra IJ (1976 a) An assessment of daily turnover and significance of thyroidal secretion of reverse T_3. J Clin Invest 58:32

Chopra IJ (1976 b) Radioimmunoassay of iodothyronines. Dekker, New York, Handbook of radioimmunoassay, p 679)

Chopra IJ (1977) A study of extrathyroidal conversion of thyroxine (T_4) to 3,3′,5-triiodothyronine (T_3) in vitro. Endocrinology 101:453

Chopra IJ (1978 a) Nature, source and biologic significance of thyroid hormone in blood. In: Werner SC, Ingbar SH (eds) The thyroid, 4th ed. Harper & Row, New York, p 100

Chopra IJ (1978 b) Sulfhydryl groups and monodeiodination of thyroxine to triiodothyronine. Science 199:904

Chopra IJ, Crandall BF (1975) Thyroid hormones and thyrotropin in amniotic fluid. N Engl J Med 293:740

Chopra IJ, Smith SR (1975) Circulating thyroid hormones and thyrotropin in adult patients with protein – calorie malnutrition. J Clin Endocrinol Metab 40:221 (1975)

Chopra IJ, Solomon DH (1972) Triiodothyronine in health and disease. Excerpta Med Int Congr Ser 273:1163

Chopra IJ, Solomon DH (1976) Thyroid function tests and their alterations by drugs. Pharmacol Ther [C] 1:367

Chopra IJ, Solomon DH (1979) Reduced outer ring and normal inner ring monodeiodination of iodothyronines in the fasting rat: effect of reduced nonprotein sulfhydryl groups (NP-SH) and hypothyroidism. Clin Res 27:19 A

Chopra IJ, Dussault JH, Fisher DA, Solomon DH (1971 a) The sources of circulating triiodothyronine (T_3) in man. Clin Res 19:560

Chopra IJ, Solomon DH, Beall GN (1971 b) Radioimmunoassay for measurement of triiodothyronine in human serum. J Clin Invest 50:2033

Chopra IJ, Nelson JC, Solomon DH, Beall GN (1971 c) Production of antibodies specifically binding triiodothyronine and thyroxine. J Clin Endocrinol Metab 32:299

Chopra IJ, Ho RS, Lam R (1972 a) An improved radioimmunoassay of triiodothyronine in serum: its application to clinical and physiological studies. J Lab Clin Med 80:729 (1972 a).

Chopra IJ, Solomon DH, Ho RS (1972 b) Competitive ligand binding assay for measurement of thyroxine binding globulin (TBG). J Clin Endocrinol Metab 35:565

Chopra IJ, Solomon DH, Chua Teco GN (1973 a) Thyroxine: just a prohormone or a hormone too? J Clin Endocrinol Metab 36:1050

Chopra IJ, Fisher DA, Solomon DH (1973 b) Thyroxine and triiodothyronine in the human thyroid. J Clin Endocrinol Metab 36:311

Chopra IJ, Solomon DH, Chopra U, Young RT, Chua Teco GN (1974) Alterations in circulating thyroid hormones and thyrotropin in hepatic cirrhosis: evidence for euthyroidism despite subnormal serum triiodothyronine. J Clin Endocrinol Metab 39:501

Chopra IJ, Sack J, Fisher DA (1975 a) Circulating 3,3′,5′-triiodothyronine in the human newborn. J Clin Invest 55:1137

Chopra IJ, Sack J, Fisher DA (1975 b) 3,3′,5′-triiodothyronine (reverse T_3) in fetal and adult sheep: studies of metabolic clearance rate, production rate, serum binding and thyroidal content relative to thyroxine. Endocrinology 97:1080

Chopra IJ, Williams DE, Orgiazzi J, Solomon DH (1975 c) Opposite effects of dexamethasone on serum concentrations of 3,3′,5′-triiodothyronine (reverse T_3) and 3,3′,5-triiodothyronine (T_3). J Clin Endocrinol Metab 41:911

Chopra IJ, Chopra U, Smith SR, Reza M, Solomon DH (1975 d) Reciprocal changes in serum concentrations of 3,3′,5′-triiodothyronine (reverse T_3) and 3,3′,5-triiodothyronine (T_3) in systematic illnesses. J Clin Endocrinol Metab 41:1043

Chopra IJ, Hershman JM, Hornabrook RW (1975 e) A study of serum thyroid hormone and thyrotropin levels in subjects from endemic goiter regions of New Guinea. J Clin Endocrinol Metab 40:326

Chopra IJ, Wu SY, Nakamura Y, Solomon DH (1978 a) Monodeiodination of 3,5,3'-triiodothyronine (T_3) and 3,3',5'-triiodothyronine (reverse T_3) to 3,3'-diiodothyronine (T_2) in vitro. Endocrinology 102:1099

Chopra IJ, Carlson HE, Solomon DH (1978 b) Comparison of the effects of 3,5,3'-triiodothyronine (T_3), thyroxine (T_4), 3,3',5'-triiodothyronine (reverse T_3) and 3,3'-diiodothyronine (T_2) on thyrotropin – releasing hormone induced release of thyrotropin in the rat in vitro. Endocrinology 103:393

Chopra IJ, Solomon DH, Chopra U, Wu SY, Fisher DA, Nakamura Y (1978 c) Pathways of metabolism of thyroid hormones. Recent Prog Horm Res 34:521

Chopra IJ, Geola F, Solomon DH, Maciel RMB (1978 d) 3'5'-diiodothyronine in health and disease: studies by a radioimmunoassay. J Clin Endocrinol Metab 47:1198

Chopra IJ, Solomon DH, Hepner GW, Morgenstein A (1979 a) Misleadingly low free T_4 index (FT_4I) and usefulness of reverse T_3 (rT_3) measurement in nonthyroidal illnesses. Ann Intern Med 90:905

Chopra IJ, Chua Teco GN, Nguyen AH, Solomon DH (1979 b) In search of inhibitor of thyroid hormone binding to serum proteins in nonthyroid illnesses. J Clin Endocrinol Metab 49:63

Cilento G (1975) In deference of a special role for the iodo substituents in thyroid hormones. J Theor Biol 52:255

Cilento G, Berenholc M (1965) Heavy-atom pertubation, molecular complexing and activity of thyroxine. Biochem Biophys Acta 94:271

Clark JH, Klee W, Levitzki A, Wolff J (eds) (1976) Hormone and antihormone action at the target cell. Dahlem Konferenzen, Berlin

Cody V (1974) Crystal structure and molecular conformation of the thyroid hormone distal 3,5,3'-triiodo-L-thyronine. J Am Chem Soc 96:6720

Cody V (1975) Distal conformation of thyroid hormones. Crystal and molecular structure of 3,5,3'-triiodo-L-thyronine methyl ester. J Med Chem 18:126

Cody V (1976) Conformational characteristics of thyroid hormones: Structure-function relationships and hormone binding. In: Robbins J, Braverman LE (eds) Thyroid research. Excerpta Medica, New York, p 290

Cody V (1978 a) Thyroid hormones: crystal structure, molecular conformation, binding, and structure-function relationships. Recent Progr Horm Res 34:437

Cody V (1978 b) Molecular conformation of a halogen-free thyroxine analogue: 4'-methoxy-3,5,3'-trimethyl-L-thyronine N-acetyl ethyl ester. Science 201:1131

Cody V, Hazel JP (1976) Molecular structures of thyroxine analogues: the crystal structures of tetraiodothyroacetic acid and tetraiodo-thyroformic acid N-diethanolamine complexes. Am Crystallogr Assoc Meet, abstract PA 6

Cody V, Hazel JP (1977) An accurate molecular determination of thyroxine. abstract PB1 Am Crystallogr Assoc Meet.

Cody V, Duax WL, Norton DA (1972) Molecular conformation of the thyroxine analogue 3,5-diiodo-L-thyronine N-methylacetamide complex (1 : 1). Acta Crystallogr B28:2244

Cody V, Duax WL, Hauptman HA (1973) Conformational analysis of aromatic amino acids by X-ray crystallography. Int J Pept Protein Res 5:297

Cody V, Erman M, DeJarnette FE (1975) Molecular structures of thyroxine analogues: the crystal structures of 3,5-dibromothyroacetic acid and 3,5-diiodothyropropionic acid. Am Crystallogr Assoc Meet, abstract H1

Cody V, Erman M, DeJarnette FE (1977 a) Crystal structure of the active thyroxine analogue, 3,5-diiodothyropropionic acid [3- (4-hydroxyphenoxy-3,5-diiodophenyl) propanoic acid]. J Chem Res 126 S. 126

Cody V, Hazel JP, Langs DA, Duax WL (1977 b) Molecular structure of thyroxine analogues: crystal structure of 3,5,3'-triiodothyroacetic and 3,5,3',5'-tetraiodothyroacetic acid N-diethanolamine (1 : 1) complexes. J Med Chem 20:1628

Cody V, Hazel JP, Osawa Y (1978) 3,5,3'-triiodo-4'-methoxythyropropionic acid methyl ester. Acta Cryst allogr B34:3407

Cody V, Podolski M, Niebor E, Falter H (1974) Solid state and solution conformation of thyroid hormones. MEDI. Am Chem Soc Meet, abstract 76

Cortell RE (1949) The antithyroxine activity of thyroxine analogues. J Clin Endocrinol Metab 9:955

Croxson M, Ibbertson IM (1977) Low serum triiodothyronine (T_3) and hypothyroidism in anorexia nervosa. J Clin Endocrinol Metab 44:167

Croxson MS, Hall TD, Nicoloff JT (1977) Combination drug therapy for treatment of hyperthyroid Graves' disease. J Clin Endocrinol Metab 45:623

Danforth E jr, Sims EAH, Horton ES, Colman RF (1975) Correlation of serum triiodothyronine concentrations (T_3) with dietary composition, gain in weight and thermogenesis in man. Diabetes [Suppl 2] 24:406

Danforth E jr, Tyzibir ED, Horton ES, Sims EAH, Burger AG, Braverman LE, Vagenakis AG, Ingbar SH (1976) Reciprocal changes in serum triiodothyronine (T_3) and reverse T_3 (rT_3) induced by altering the carbohydrate content of the diet. Clin Res 24:271A

Davidson MB, Chopra IJ (1979) Effect of carbohydrate and noncarbohydrate sources of calories on plasma T_3 concentration in man. J Clin Endocrinol Metab 48:577

Davis PJ, Handwerger BS, Gregerman RI (1972) Thyroid hormone binding by human serum prealbumin (TBPA). Electrophoretic studies of triiodothyronine TBPA interaction. J. Clin Invest 51:515

DeGroot LJ, Haye K (1976) Dexamethasone suppression of serum T_3 and T_4. J Clin Endocrinol Metab 42:976

DeGroot LJ, Torresani J (1975) Triiodothyronine binding to isolated liver cell nuclei. Endocrinology 96:357

DeLange F, Camus M, Ermans AM (1972) Circulating thyroid hormones in endemic goiter. J Clin Endocrinol Metab 34:891

Dianik N, Hoffman R, Maffei LA, Forget BC (1978) Potentiation of human erythropoiesis in vitro by thyroid hormone. Nature 272:260

Dietrich SW (1976) Thyroid hormone analogs: synthesis, thyromimetic activities molecular orbital studies, and quantitative structure-activity correlations. PhD thesis, University of California

Dietrich SW, Bolger MB, Kollman PA, Jorgensen EC (1977) Thyroxine analogues. 23. Quantitative structure-activity correlation studies of in vivo and in vitro thyromimetic activities. J Med Chem 20:863

Dowling JT, Freinkel N, Ingbar SH (1956) Thyroxine binding by sera of pregnant women, newborn infants and women with spontaneous abortion. J Clin Invest 35:1263

Duick DS, Warren DW, Nicoloff JT, Otis CL, Croxson MS (1974) Effect of single dose dexamethasone on the concentration of serum triiodothyronine in man. J Clin Endocrinol Metab 39:1151

Dunn JT, Stanbury JB (1958) The metabolism of 3:3′:5′-triiodothyronine in man. J Clin Endocrinol Metab 18:713

Dussault JH, Lam R, Fisher DA (1971) The measurement of serum triiodothyronine by double column chromatography. J Lab Clin Med 77:1039

Eisenstein Z, Hagg S, Vagenakis AG, Fang SL, Ransil B, Burger A, Braverman LE, Ingbar SH (1978) Effect of starvation on the production and peripheral metabolism of 3,3′,5′-triiodothyronine in euthyroid obese subjects. J Clin Endocrinol Metab 47:889

Ekins RP, In Sterling K (1970) The significance of circulating triiodothyronine. Recent Progr Horm Res 26:283

Emmett JC, Pepper ES (1975) Conformation of thyroid hormone analogues. Nature 257:334

Engler D, Merkelbach U, Burger AG (1979) Further characterization of the monodeiodination of triiodothyronine (T_3) by radioimmunoassay of 3,5-diiodothyronine (3,5-T_2). Clin Res 27:251

Engstrom WW, Markardt B (1954) Influence of estrogen on thyroid function. J Clin Endocrinol Metab 14:215

Engstrom WW, Markardt B, Liebman A (1952) Effect of estrogens on serum precipitable iodine. Proc Soc Exp Biol Med 81:582

Erenberg A, Phelps D, Lam RW, Fisher DA (1974) Total and free thyroxine and triiodothyronine concentrations in the newborn period. Pediatrics 53:211

Faber J, Kirkegaard BC, Ragowski P, Siersback-Nielsen K, Friis T (1978) Urinary excretion of 3,3′,5′-triiodothyronine (reverse T_3). Clin Endocrinol (Oxf) 9:279

Fang VS, Lim VS, Refetoff S (1974) Triiodothyronine (T_3) hypothyroidism in patients with renal in sufficiency. Ann Meet Am Thyroid Assoc T-16

Farer LS, Robins J, Blumberg BS, Rall JE (1962) Thyroxine-serum protein complexes in various animals. Endocrinology 70:686

Fawcett JK, Camerman N, Camerman A (1976 a) Thyroid hormone stereochemistry. IV. Molecular conformation of 3′-isopropyl-3,5-diiodo-L-thyronine in the crystal and in solution. J Am Chem Soc 98:587

Fawcett JK, Camerman N, Camerman A (1976 b) Structure of 2′,3′-dimethyl-3,5-diiodo-DL-thyronine; a fixed-conformation analogue of the thyroid hormone 3,5,3′-triiodo-L-thyronine. Can J Chem 54:1317

Ferguson DC, Jennings AS, Utiger RD (1979) Conversion of thyroxine (T_4) to triiodothyronine (T_3) in the perfused rat kidney. Clin Res 27:251A

Fisher DA, Dussault DH (1971) Contribution of methodologic artifacts to the measurement of T_3 concentration in serum. J Clin Endocrinol Metab 32:675

Fisher DA, Dussault JH (1974) thyroid. In: Greer MA, Solomon DH (eds) Endocrinology III. The Williams & Wilkins, Baltimore, Handbook of physiology; p 21)

Fisher DA, Oddie TH (1964) Whole body counting of ^{131}I-labeled triiodothyronine. J Clin Endocrinol Metab 24:733

Fisher DA, Odell WD (1969) Acute release of thyrotropin in the newborn. J Clin Invest 48:1670

Fisher DA, Chopra IJ, Dussault JH (1972) Extrathyroidal conversion of thyroxine to triiodothyronine in the sheep. Endocrindogy 91:1141

Fisher DA, Dussault JH, Sack J, Chopra IJ (1977) Ontogenesis of hypothalamo – pituitary – thyroid function and metabolism in man, sheep and rat. Recent Prog Horm Res 33:59

Fisher DA, Sack J, Oddie TH, Pekary AE, Hersman JM, Lam RW, Parslow ME (1978) Serum T_4, TBG, T_3 uptake, T_3, reserve T_3, and TSH concentrations in children 1 to 15 years of age. J Clin Endocrinol Metab 45:191

Fishman N, Huang YP, Tergis DC, Rivlin RS (1977) Relation of triiodothyronine and reverse triiodothyronine adminstration in rats to hepatic L-triiodothyronine aminotransferase activity. Endocrinology 100:1055

Freinkel N, Ingbar SH, Dowling JP (1957) The influence of extracellular thyroxine binding protein upon the accumulation of thyroxine by tissue slices. J Clin Invest 36:25

Gaddum JH (1930) Quantitative observations on thyroxine and allied substances. II. Effects on the oxygen consumption of rats. J Physiol (Lond) 68:383

Galasso V, DeAlti G, Bigotto A (1971) The conformation of diphenyl ether, sulphide and selenide. A quantum-mechanical interpretation. Tetrahedron 27:6151

Galton VA (1976) The metabolism of thyroid hormones in rat pituitary. In: Braverman LE (ed), Thyroid research. Excerpta Medica, Amsterdam, p 251

Galton VA, Pitt-Rivers R (1959). The identification of the acetic acid analogues of thyroxine and triiodothyronine in mamalian tissues. Biochem J 72:319

Gardner DF, Kaplan MM, Stanley CS, Utiger RD (1979) The effect of T_3 replacement on the metabolic and pituitary responses to starvation. N Engl J Med 300:579

Gavin LA, Rosenthal M (1977) Thyroxine pseudtoxicosis: a compensatory response in nonthyroid systemic illness. Annu Meet Amer Thyroid Assoc p. T-4.

Gavin L, Castle J, McMahon F, Martin P, Hammond M, Cavalieri R (1977) Extrathyroidal conversion of thyroxine to 3,3′,5′-triiodothyronine (reverse T_3) and to 3,5,3′-triiodothyronine (T_3) in humans. J Clin Endocrinol Metab 44:133

Gavin LA, Hammond ME, Castle JN, Cavalieri RR (1978) 3,3′-diiodothyronine, a major pathway of peripheral iodothyronine metabolism in man. J Clin Invest 61:1276

Geffner DL, Azukikawa M, Hershaman J (1975) Propylthiouracil blocks extrathyroidal conversion of thyroxine to triiodothyronine and augments thyrotropin secretion in man. J Clin Invest 55:224

Geola F, Chopra IJ, Solomon DH, Maciel RMB (1979) Metabolic clearance and production rates of 3′,5′-diiodothyronine (3′,5′-T_2) and 3,3′-diiodothyronine (3,3′-T_2) in man. J Clin Endocrinol Metab 48:297

Gharib H, Mayberry WE, Ryan RJ (1970) Radioimmunoassay for triiodothyronine: a preliminary report. J Clin Endocrinol Metab 31:709

Gharib H, Ryan RJ, Mayberry WE, Hockert T (1971) Radioimmunoassay for triiodothyronine (T_3): I. Affinity and specificity of the antibody for T_3. J Clin Endocrinol Metab 33:509

Giorgio NA, jr, Tabachnik M (1968) Thyroxine protein interactions. V. Isolation and characterization of a thyroxine binding globulin from human plasma. J Biol Chem 243:2247

Gley E, Bourcet P (1900) Présence de l'iode dans le sang. CR Acad Sci [D] (Paris) 130:1721

Glinoer D, Gershengorn MC, Dubois A, Robbins J (1977) Stimulation of thyroxine binding globulin synthesis by isolated rhesus monkey hepatocytes after in vitro β-estradiol administration. Endocrinology 100:807

Golde DW, Bersch N, Chopra IJ, Cline MJ (1977) Thyroid hormones stimulate erythropoiesis in vitro. Br J Haematol 37:173

Goldfine ID, Simons CG, Ingbar SH (1975) Stimulation of the uptake of α-aminoisobutyric acid in rat thymocytes by L-triiodothyronine: a comparison with insulin and dibutyryl cyclic AMP. Endocrinology 96:802

Goldfine ID, Smith GJ, Simons CG, Ingbar JH, Jorgensen EC (1976) Activities of thyroid hormones and related compounds in an in vitro thymocyte assay. J Biol Chem 251:4233
Goldman RF, Haisman MF, Bynum G, Danforth E jr, Horton ES, Sims EAH (1975) Experimental obesity in man. Metabolic rate in relation to dietary intake. In: Bray GA (ed) Obesity in perspective, (Fogarty International Center Series on Preventive Medicine, U. S. Government Printing Office, Washington, D.C. p 165)
Gordon AH, Gross J, O'Connor D, Pitt-Rivers R (1952) Nature of the circulating thyroid hormone-plasma protein complex. Nature 169:19
Graves RJ (1835) Clinical lectures. London Med Surg J 7:516
Green JRB, Smitcher EJ, Mowat NAG, Ekins RP, Rees LH, Dawson AM (1977) Thyroid function and thyroid regulation in euthyroid man with chronic liver disease: evidence of multiple abnormalities. Clin Endocrinol (Oxf) 7:453
Green WL (1976) Thyroxine metabolism by rat liver slices: evidence for a specific T_3-forming pathway. In: Robbins J, Braverman LE (eds) Thyroid research. Excerpta Medica, Amsterdam, p 239
Greenberg AH, Czernichow P, Reba RC, Tyson J, Blizzard RM (1970) Observations on the maturation of thyroid function in early fetal life. J Clin Invest 49:1790
Greenberg CM, Blank B, Pfeiffer FR, Pauls JF (1963) Relative activities of several 3'- and 3',5'-alkyl and aryl thyromimetic agents. Am J Physiol 205:821
Greer MA (1951) Evidence of hypothalamic control of the pituitary release of thyrotropin. Proc Soc Exp Biol Med 77:603
Gregerman RI, Solomon N (1967) Acceleration of thyroxine and triiodothyronine turnover during bacterial pulmonary injections and fever: implications for the functional state of the thyroid during stress and in senescence. J Clin Endocrinol Metab 27:93
Grinberg R, Volpert EM, Werner SC (1963) In vivo deiodination of labeled L-thyroxine to L-3,5,3'-triiodothyronine in mouse and human pituitaries. J Clin Endocrinol Metab 23:140
Gross J, Leblond CP (1951) The presence of free iodinated compounds in the thyroid and their passage in the circulation. Endocrinology 48:714
Gross J, Pitt-Rivers R (1952) The identification 3,5,3'-triiodothyronine in human plasma. Lancet I:439
Gross J, Pitt-Rivers R (1953) 3,5,3'-triiodothyronine. 1. Isolation from thyroid gland and synthesis. Biochem J 53:645
Gross J, Leblond CP, Franklin AE, Onastel JH (1950) Presence of iodinated amino acids in unhydrolyzed thyroid and plasma. Science 111:605
Grussendorf M, Ntokalau M, Hufner M (1977) Pathways of thyroxine monodeiodination in rat liver homogenate. Acta Endocrinol (Copenh) [Suppl 208] 84:16
Gull WW (1874) On a cretinoid state supervening in adult life in women. Trans Clin Soc (Lond) 7:180
Hagen GA, Dinguid LI, Kliman B, Stanbury JB (1970) Double-isotope derivative assay of serum iodothyronines. I. Preparation of acetyl derivatives of thyroxine and triiodothyronine. Anal Biochem 33:67
Hagen GA, Diguid LI, Kliman B, Stanbury JB (1973) Double isotope derivative assay of serum iodothyronines. 3. Triiodothyronine. Biochem Med 7:191.
Hagg S, Popitz M, Ingbar SH (1978) In vitro inhibitory effect of reverse triiodothyronine (rT_3) on lipolysis in rat adipocytes. Annu Meet Amer. Thyroid Assoc., p. T-20
Haibach H (1971) Free iodothyronines in the rat thyroid gland. Endocrinology 88:149
Hao Y, Tabachnick M (1971) Thyroxine-protein interactions. VII. Effect of ^{125}I-thyroxine to highly purified human thyroxine-binding globulin. Endocrinology 28:81
Harrington CR (1926) Chemistry of thyroxine. I. Isolation of thyroxine from thyroid gland. Biochem J 20:293
Harrington CR (1933) The thyroid gland: Its chemistry and physiology. Oxford University Press, London
Harrington CR, Barger G (1927) Chemistry of thyroxine. III Constitution of synthesis of thyroxine. Biochem J 21:169
Harris ARC, Fang SL, Prosky J, Braverman LE, Vagenakis AG (1978) Decreased outer ring monodeiodination of thyroxine and reverse triiodothyronine in the fetal and neonatal rat. Endocrinology 103:2216
Harris A, Fang S, Braverman L, Vagenakis A (1979) The role of sulfhydryl groups (SH) on the impaired hepatic 3',3,5-triiodothyronine generation from thyroxine in the hypothyroid, starved, fetal and neonatal rodent. J Clin Invest 63:516

Heinemann M, Johnson CE, Man EB (1948) The serum-precipitable iodine concentrations during pregnancy. J Clin Invest 27:91

Hershman JM, Pittman JR jr (1970) Response to synthetic thyrotropin-releasing hormone in man. J Clin Endocrinol Metab 31:457

Hesch RD, Grunner G, Soling D (1975) Conversion of thyroxine (T_4) to triiodothyronine and subcellular localization of the converting enzyme. Clin Chim Acta 59:209

Hesch RD, Gatz J, Pope J, Schmidt E, Zur Muhlen A von (1976) Total and free triiodothyronine and thyroid binding globulin concentration in elderly human persons. Eur J Clin Invest 6:139

Higasi K, Smyth CP (1960) Microwave absorption and molecular structure. XXXIII. Change in mesomeric moment as a mechanism of dielectric relation. J Am Chem Soc 82:4759

Hollander CS (1968) On the nature of circulating thyroid hormone: Clinical studies of triiodothyronine and thyroxine in serum using gas chromatographic methods. Trans Assoc Am Physicians 81:76

Hollander CS, Mitsuma F, Nihei N, Shenkman L, Burday SZ, Blum M (1972) Clinical and laboratory observations in cases of triiodothyronine toxicosis confirmed by radioimmunoassay. Lancet I:609

Holm AC, Jorgensen EC, Pliam NB, Goldfine ID (1977) Membrane transport and cellular effects of thyroid hormones. Ann Endocrinol (Paris) 38: abstract 103

Hoskins RG (1949) The thyroid–pituitary apparatus as a servo (feed-back) mechanism. J Clin Endocrinol Metab 9:1429

Hufner M, Hesch RD (1973) Triiodothyronine determinations in urine. Lancet I:101

Hufner M, Knopfle M (1976) Pharmacological influences on T_4 to T_3 conversion in rat liver. Clin Chim Acta 72:337

Hufner M, Grussendorf M, Ntokalou M (1977) Properties of the thyroxine (T_4) monodeiodinating system in rat liver homogenate. Clin Chim Acta 78:251

Inada M, Kasagi K, Kurata S, Kazama Y, Takayama H, Torizuka K, Fukase M, Soma T (1975) Estimation of thyroxine and triiodothyronine distribution and of the conversion rate of thyroxine to triiodothyronine in man. J Clin Invest 55:1337

Ingbar SH (1958) Prealbumin: a thyroxine-binding protein of human plasma. Endocrinology 63:256

Ingbar SH (1963) Observations concerning the binding of thyroid hormones by human serum prealbumin. J Clin Invest 42:163

Ingbar SH, Freinkel N (1955) Simultaneous estimation of rates of thyroxine degradation and thyroid hormone synthesis. J Clin Invest 34:808

Ingbar SH, Freinkel N (1960) Regulation of the peripheral metabolism of the thyroid hormones. Recent Progr Horm Res 16:353

Ingenbleek Y, de Visscher M, de Nayer PH (1972) Measurement of prealbumin as index of protein-calorie malnutrition. Lancet II: 106

Izumi M, Larsen PR (1977) Triiodothyronine, thyroxine and iodine in purified thyroglobulin from patients with Graves' disease. J Clin Invest 59:1105

Jorgensen EC (1964) Stereochemistry of thyroxine and analogs. Mayo Clin Proc 39:560

Jorgensen EC (1976) Structure activity relationships of thyroxine analogues. Pharmacol Ther [B] 2:661

Jorgensen EC (1978) Thyroid hormone structure-function relationships. In: Werner SC, Ingbar SH (eds) The thyroid, 4th ed. Harper & Row, New York

Jorgensen EC, Lehmann PA, Greenberg C, Zenker N (1962) Thyroxine analogues. VII. Antigoitrogenic, calorigenic, and hypocholestesteremic activities of some aliphatic, alicyclic, and aromatic ehters of 3,5-diiodothyronine in the rat. J Biol Chem 237:3832

Jorgensen EC, Murray WJ, Block P jr (1974) Thyroxine analogs. 22. Thyromimetic activity of halogen-free derivatives of 3,5-dimethyl-L-thyronine. J Med Chem 17:434

Kalant H, Lee R, Sellers EA (1955) Metabolic fate of radioactive thyroid hormones in normal and propylthiouracil-treated rats. Endocrinology 56:127

Kanda Y, Goodman DS, Canfield RE, Morgan FJ (1974) The amino acid sequence of human plasma prealbumin. J Biol Chem 249: 6796

Kaplan MM (1978) T_4 to T_3 conversion in rat pituitary homogenate. Annu Meet Amer Thyroid Assoc. p T-6

Kaplan MM, Utiger RD (1978 a) Iodothyronine metabolism in rat liver homogenates. J Clin Invest 61:459

Kaplan MM, Utiger RD (1978 b) Iodothyronine metabolism in liver and kidney homogenates from hyperthyroid and hypothyroid rats. Endocrinology 103:156

Kaplan MM, Schimmel M, Utiger RD (1977) Changes in serum 3,3',5'-triiodothyronine (reverse T_3) concentrations with altered thyroid hormone secretion and metabolism. J Clin Endocrinol Metab 45:447

Kendall EC (1915) The isolation in crystalline form of the compound containing iodine which occurs in the thyroid: its chemical nature and physiological activity. Trans Assoc Am Physicians 30:420

Kier LB, Hoyland JR (1970) A molecular orbital study of 3,3',5-trihalothyronine analogs. J Med Chem 13:1182

Klein AH, Oddie TH, Fisher DA (1978) Effect of parturition on serum iodothyronine concentrations in fetal sheep. Endocrinology 103:1453

Klotz IM (1973) Physicochemical aspects of drug-protein interactions: a general perspective. Ann NY Acad Sci 226:18

Klyne W, Prelog V (1960) Description of steric relationships across single bonds. Experientia 56:521

Kocher T (1883) Über Kropfexstirpation und ihre Folgen. Arch Klin Chir 29:254

Kochupillai N, Deo MG, Karmarkar MG, McKendrick M, Weightman D, Evered DC, Hall R, Ramalinga-swamy V (1973) Pituitary thyroid axis in Himalayan endemic goiter. Lancet 1:1021

Koerner D, Surks MI, Oppenheimer JH (1974) In vitro demonstration of specific triiodothyronine binding sites in rat liver nuclei. J Clin Endocrinol Metab 38:706

Koerner D, Schwartz HL, Surks MI, Oppenheimer JH, Jorgensen EC (1975) Binding of selected iodothyronine analogues to receptor sites of isolated rat hepatic nuclei: high correlation between structural requirements for nuclear binding and biologic activity. J Biol Chem 250:6417

Kollman PA, Murray WJ, Nuss ME, Jorgensen EC, Rothenberg S (1973) Molecular orbital studies of thyroid hormone analogs. J Am Chem Soc 95:8518

Korcek L, Tabachnick M (1976) Thyroxine-protein interactions. Interaction of thyroxine and triiodothyronine with human thyroxine-binding globulin. J Biol Chem 251:3558

Koutras DA, Berman M, Sfontouris J, Rigopoulos GA, Koukoulommati AS, Malamos B (1970) Endemic goiter in Greece: thyroid hormone kinetics. J Clin Endocrinol Metab 30:479

Kubinyi H (1976) Quantitative structure-activity relationships. 2. A mixed approach, based on Hansch and Free-Wilson analysis. J Med Chem 19:587

Larsen PR (1971) Inhibition of triiodothyronine (T_3) binding to thyroxine binding globulin by sodium salicylate and its application to immunoassay of T_3 in human serum. Metabolism 20:976

Larsen PR (1972a) Salicylate-induced increases in free triiodo-thyronine in human serum. Evidence of inhibition of triiodothyronine binding to thyroxine binding globulin and thyroxine binding prealbumin J Clin Invest 51:1125

Larsen PR (1972b) Triiodothyronine: review of recent studies of its physiology and pathophysiology in man. Metabolism 21:1073

Larsen PR (1972c) Direct immunoassay of triiodothyronine in human serum. J Clin Invest 51:1939

Larsen PR, Yamashita K, Dekker A, Field JB (1973) Biochemical observations in functioning human thyroid adenomas. J Clin Endocrinol Metab 36:1009

Larson FC, Albright EC (1961) Inhibition of L-thyroxine monodeiodination by thyroxine analogs. J Clin Invest 40:1132

Larson FC, Deiss WP, Albright EC (1952) Localization of protein-bound radioactive iodine by filter paper electrophoresis. Science 115:626

Lassiter WC, Stanbury JB (1958) The in vivo conversion of thyroxine to 3, 5, 3'-triiodothyronine. J Clin Endocrinol Metab 18:903

Latham KR, Ring JC, Baxter JD (1976) Solubilized nuclear "receptors" for thyroid hormones. J Biol Chem 23:7388

Laurberg P (1978) Nonparallel variations in the preferential secretion of 3,5,3'-triiodothyronine (T_3) and 3,3',5'-triiodothyronine (rT_3) from dog thyroid. Endocrinology 102:757

Laurberg P, Weeke J (1978) Opposite variations in serum T_3 and reverse T_3 during prophythiouracil treatment of thyrotoxicosis. Acta Endocrinol (Copenh) 87:88

Lehmann PA (1972) Intramolecular aryl-iodine π complex formation and its relation to thyromimetic activity. J Med Chem 15:404

Lehmann PA, (1974) Stereoelectronic factors in the submolecular mode of action of thyromimetics. Intra Sci Chem Rep 8:117

Lehmann PA, Jorgensen EC (1965) Thyroxine analogs-XIII. NMR evidence for hindered rotation in diphenyl ethers. Tetrahedron 21:363

Lemarchand – Beraud T, Holm AC, Bornand G, Burger A (1978) High affinity binding of reverse T_3 and tetrac in nuclei of human lymphocytes. Acta Endocrinol (Copenh) 87:516

Leonard JL, Rosenberg IN (1978) Subcellular distribution of thyroxine 5′-deiodinase in the rat kidney, a plasma membrane location. Endocrinology 103:274

Leonard JL, Rosenberg IN (1979) Interactions of 6-n-propyl-2-thiouracil and T_4 5′-deiodinase. Annu Meet Endocr Soc, abstract 661, p 238

Levey G, Epstein SE (1969) Myocardial adenyl cyclase: activation by thyroid hormones and evidence for two adenyl cyclase systems. J Clin Invest 48:1663

Levy RP, Marshall JS, Velayo NL (1971) Radioimmunoassay of human thyroxine binding globulin (TBG). J Clin Endocrinol Metab 32:373

Lieblich J, Utiger RD (1972) Triiodothyronine radioimmunoassay. J Clin Invest 51:157

Livermore BM, Gavin LA, Castle JN, Hammond ME, Cavalieri RR (1979) Serum concentration, metabolic clearance and turnover rates of triac in normal and athyreotic man. Annu Meet Endocr Soc, abstract 76, p 91

Lo C-S, Edelman IS (1976) Effect of triiodothyronine on the synthesis and degradation of renal cortical $(Na^+ + K^+)$ – adenosine triphosphatase. J Biol Chem 251:7834

Maciel RMB, Ozawa Y, Chopra IJ (1979a) Subcellular localization of thyroxine and reverse triiodothyronine outer ring monodeiodinating activities. Endocrinology 104:365

Maciel RMB, Chopra IJ, Ozawa Y, Geola F, Solomon DH (1979b) A radioimmunoassay for measurement of 3,5-diiodothyronine (3,5-T_2). J Clin Endocrinol Metab 48:399

Maclagan NF, Boweden CH, Wilkinson JH, (1957) The metabolism of thyroid hormones. II. Detection of thyroxine and triiodothyronine in human plasma. Biochem J 67:5

Magnus-Levy A, (1895) Über den respiratorischen Gaswechsel unter dem Einfluß der Thyroidea Säure unter verschiedenen pathologischen Zuständen. Klin Wochenschr 32:650

Maguire SB, Dennehy A, Cullen MJ (1976) The effect of thyrotoxicosis and hypothyroidism on the extrathyroidal conversion of thyroxine to triiodothyronine in man. In: Robbins J, Braverman L (eds) Thyroid research. Excerpta Medica, Amsterdam, p 259

Mandel LR, Kuehl FA (1967) Lipolytic action of 3,3′,5-triiodo-L-thyronine. Biochem Biophys Res Commun 28:13

Marcus R (1975) Cyclic nucleotide phosphodiesterase from bone: characterization of the enzyme and studies of inhibition by thyroid hormones. Endocrinology 96:400

Marcus R, Lundquist C, Chopra IJ (1975) In vitro inhibition of cyclic nucleotide phosphodiesterase (PDE) by thyroid hormones. Clin Res 23:94 A

Marshall JS, Pensky J (1969) Studies on human thyroxine binding globulin (TBG). I. Purification of TBG and immunologic studies on the relationship between TBG from normal persons and those with TBG "deficiency". J Clin Invest 48:508

Marshall JS, Williams S, Jones P, Hepner GW (1978) Serum desialylated glycoproteins in patients with hepatobiliary dysfunction. J Lab Clin Med 92:30

Mauchamp J, Shinitzky M (1969) The nature of thyroxine and related compounds as electron donors. Biochemistry 8:1554

Mazzocchi PH, Ammon HL, Colicelli E, Hohokabe Y, Cody V (1976) NMR-studies of triiodothyropropionic acid in ethanol-HCl. Experientia 32:419

McLarty DC, Ratcliffe WA, McCall K, Stone D, Ratcliffe JG (1975) Thyroid hormone levels and prognosis in patients with serious nonthyroid illness. Lancet II: 275

Means JH (1954) The thyroid hormone- certain aspects of its elaboration in the body, the significance of its structure and of its action on end organs. In: Lectures on the thyroid, Harvard University Press, Cambridge, pp 21–40

Medeiros-Neto GA, Sucupira M, Knobel M, Cinbia AU (1977) Prolactin, TSH and thyroid hormones, responses to TRH in adult protein calorie malnutrition. Horm Metab Res 9:524

Medeiros-Neto GA, Walfish PG, Almeida F, Maia E, Gomes E, Kiy Y, Knobel M, Ginsberg J, Chopra IJ (1978) 3,3′5′-triiodothyronine, thyroxine, triiodothyronine and thyrotropin levels in maternal and cord blood sera from endemic goiter regions of Brazil. J Clin Endocrinol Metab 47:508

Meinhold H, Schurnabrand P (1978) A radioimmunoassay for 3,5-diiodothyronine. Clin Endocrinol (Oxf) 8:493

Meinhold H, Wenzel KW, Schurnabrand PZ (1975) Radioimmunoassay of L-3,3′,5′-triiodo-L-thyronine (reverse T_3) in human serum and its application in different thyroid states. Z Klin Chem Biochem 13:571

Michel R, Pitt-Rivers R, Roche J, Varrone S (1962) On the formation of 3,5,3-triiodothyracetic acid from 3,5,3-triiodo-L-thyronine. Biochem, Biophys Acta 57:335

Mitra J, Ramakrishnan C (1977) Analysis of O-H. . .O hydrogen bonds. Int J Pept Protein Res 9:27

Mitsuma T, Gershengorn JC, Hollander CS (1971) Radioimmunoassay of triiodothyronine in unextracted human serum. J Clin Endocrinol Metab 33:364
Mitsuma T, Colucci J, Shenkman L, Hollander CS (1972) Simultaneous radioimmunoassay for triiodothyronine and thyroxine in unextracted serum. Biochem Biophys Res Commun 46:2107
Miyai K, Yamamoto T, Azukikawa M, Ishibashi K, Kumahara T (1975) Serum thyroid hormones and thyrotropin in anorexia nervosa. J Clin Endocrinol Metab 40:334
Mlholm JH, Skovsted L, Siersback-Nielsen K (1975) Age dependent changes in iodine metabolism and thyroid function. Acta Endocrinol (Copenh) 79:60
Money WL, Kumaoka S, Rawson RW, Kroc RL (1960) Comparative effects of thyroxine analogues in experimental animals. Part IV. Metabolic effects of thyroid hormones and their analogues. Ann NY Acad Sci 86:512
Moshang T jr, Parks JS, Barker L, Vaidya V, Utiger RD, Bongiovanni AM, Snyder PJ (1975) Low serum triiodothyronine in patients with anorexia nervosa. J Clin Endocrinol Metab 40:470
Murphy BEP, Pattee CJ (1964) Determination of thyroxine utilizing the property of protein–binding. J Clin Endocrinol Metab 24:187
Murray WJ (1974) Thyroid hormone analogs: the role of halogen in hormonal activity. Ph D thesis, University of California
Naeije R, Clumeck N, Somers G, Vanhaelst L, Golstein J (1976) Thyroid hormones in serious non-thyroidal illness. Lancet I:1070
Nagataki S, Uchimura H, Masuyama Y, Nakao K, Itu K (1972) Triiodothyronine and thyroxine in thyroid glands of euthyroid Japanese subjects. J Clin Endocrinol Metab 35:18
Nakamura Y, Chopra IJ, Solomon DH (1977) Preparation of high specific activity radioactive iodothyronines and their analogues. J Nucl Med 18:1112
Nakamura Y, Chopra IJ, Solomon DH (1978) An assessment of the concentration of acetic acid and propionic acid derivatives of 3,5,3′-triiodothyronine in human serum. J Clin Endocrinol Metab 46:91
Naumann JA, Naumann A, Werner SC (1967) Total and free triiodothyronine in human serum. J Clin Invest 46:1346
Newcomer WS (1957) Relative potencies of thyroxine and triiodothyronine based on various criteria in thiouracil-treated chickens. Am J Physiol 190:413
Nicod P, Burger A, Staeheli V, Vallotton MB (1976) A radioimmunoassay for 3,3′,5′-triiodo-L-thyronine in unextracted serum: method and clinical results. J Clin Endocrinol Metab 42:823
Nicoloff JT, Low JC, Dussault TH, Fisher DA (1972) Simultaneous measurement of thyroxine and triiodothyronine peripheral turnover kinetics in man. J Clin Invest 51:473
Nihei N, Gershengorn, MC, Stringham LR, Cordy A, Kuchmy B, Hollander CS (1971) Measurements of triiodothyronine and thyroxine in human serum by gas liquid chromatography. Anal Biochem 43:433
Nomura S, Pittman CS, Chambers JB jr, Buck MW, Shimizu T (1975) Reduced peripheral conversion of thyroxine to triiodothyronine in patients with hepatic cirrhosis. J Clin Invest 56:643
O'Brian JT, Bybee E, Wartofsky L, Georges LP, Burman KD (1978) Altered peripheral thyroid metabolism and diminished hypothalamic pituitary responsiveness with changes in dietary composition. Clin Res 26:310A
Oddie TH, Fisher DA, Rogers C (1964) Whole body counting of ^{131}I-thyroxine. J Clin Endocrinol Metab 24:628
Oddie TH, Fisher DA, Dussault JH, Thompson CS (1971) Triiodothyronine turnover in euthyroid subjects. J Clin Endocrinol Metab 33:653
Oliver GC jr, Parker BM, Brasfield DL, Parker CW (1968) The measurement of digitoxin in human serum by radioimmunoassay. J Clin Invest 47:1035
Olsen T, Laurberg P, Weeke J (1978) Low serum triiodothyronine and high serum reverse triiodothyronine and high serum reverse triiodothyronine in old age: an effect of disease on age. J Clin Endocrinol Metab 47:1111
Oppenheimer JH, Surks MI, Bernstein G, Smith JC (1965a) Metabolism of iodine-131-labeled thyroxine-binding prealbumin in man. Science 149:748
Oppenheimer JH, Surks MI, Smith JC, Sgej R (1965b) Isolation and characterization of human thyroxine binding prealbumin. J Biol Chem 240:173
Oppenheimer JH, Martinez M, Bernstein G (1966) Determination of the maximal binding capacity and protein concentration of thyroxine binding prealbumin in human serum. J Lab Clin Med 67:500

Oppenheimer JH, Bernstein G, Hasen J (1967) Estimation of rapidly exchangeable cellular thyroxine from the plasma disappearance curves of simultaneously administered thyroxine-^{131}I and albumin-^{125}I. J Clin Inest 46:762

Oppenheimer JH, Koerner D, Schwartz HL, Surks MI (1972) Specific nuclear triiodothyronine binding sites in rat liver and kidney. J Clin Endocrinol Metab 35:330

Oppenheimer JH, Schwartz HL, Koerner D, Surks MI (1974) Limited binding capacity sites for L-triiodothyronine in rat liver nuclei. J Clin Invest 53:768

Oppenheimer JH, Schwartz HL, Surks MI (1975 a) Nuclear binding capacity appears to limit the hepatic response to L-triiodothyronine (T_3). Endocr Res Commun 2:309

Oppenheimer JH, Schwartz HL, Surks MI (1975 b) Determination of common parameters of iodothyronine metabolism and distribution in man by compartmental analysis. J Clin Endocrinol Metab 41:319

Oppenheimer JH, Schwartz HL, Surks MI (1975 c) Revised calculations of common parameters of iodothyronine metabolism and distribution by noncompartmental analysis. J Clin Endocrinol Metab 41:1172

Oppenheimer JH, Schwartz HL, Surks MI, Koerner D, Dillmann WH (1976) Nuclear receptors and the initiation of thyroid hormone action. Recent Prog Horm Res 32:529

Ord WM (1878) On myxoedema, a term proposed to be apllied to an essential condition in the "cretinoid" affection occasionally observed in middle-aged women. Med Chir Trans 61:57

Osathanondh R, Tulchinsky D, Chopra IJ (1976) Total and free triiodothyronine in normal and complicated pregnancy. J Clin Endocrinol Metab 42:98

Pangaro L, Smallridge RC, Cahnmann HJ, Wright FD, Burman KD (1979) Development of a radioimmunoassay for 3,5-diiodothyronine (3,5T_2) and demonstration of conversion from T_3. Annu Meet Endocr Soc, abstract 75, p 91

Parry CH (1825) Collections from the unpublished medical writings of the late Dr. Caleb Hilliel Parry, vol 2. Underwoods, London, p II

Patel YC, Burger HG, Morley D, Havlik H (1973 a) Simplified radioimmunoassay for triiodothyronine. J Clin Endocrinol Metab 36:187

Patel YC, Pharoah POD, Hornabrook RW, Hetzel BS (1973 b) Serum triiodothyronine, thyroxine and thyroid stimulating hormone in endemic goiter: a comparison of goitrous and nongoitrous subjects in New Guinea. J Clin Endocrinol Metab 37:783

Pauling L (1960) The nature of the chemical bond. Cornell University Press, New York, p 260

Peters JP, Man EB (1948) The relation of albumin to precipitable iodine of serum. J Clin Invest 27:397

Pharoah POD, Lawton NF, Ellis SM, Williams FS, Ekins RP (1973) The role of triiodothyronine in the maintenance of euthyroidism in endemic goitre. Clin Endocrinol (Oxf) 2:193

Pind K (1957) Paper chromatographic determination of thyroid hormone (3,5,3'-triiodothyronine) in serum without radioiodine. Acta Endocrinol (Copenh) 26:263

Piroska E, Foldes J (1976) Thyroid hormones in serious nonthyroidal illness. Lancet I:1071

Pittman CS, Chambers JB jr (1969) Carbon structure of thyroxine metabolites in urine. Endocrinology 84:705

Pittman CS, Pittman JA (1974) Relation of chemical structure to the action and metabolism of thyroactive substances. In: Greer MA, Solomon DH, (eds) Thyroid. American Physiological Society, Washington DC (Physiology, vol III) pp 233

Pittman CS, Chambers JB jr, Read VH (1971) The extrathyroidal conversion rate of thyroxine to triiodothyronine in normal man. J Clin Invest 50:1187

Pittman CS, Suda AK, Chambers JB jr, McDaniel HG, Ray GY, Preston BK (1979) Abnormalities of thyroid hormone turnover in patients with diabetes mellitus before and after insulin therapy. J Clin Endocrinol Metab 48:854

Pitt-Rivers R, Stanbury JB, Rapp B (1955) Conversion of thyroxine to 3,5,3'-triiodothyronine in vivo. J Clin Endocrinol Metab 15:616

Plaskett LG (1961) Studies on the degradation of thyroid hormones in vitro with compounds labelled in either ring. Biochem J 78:652

Ponnuswamy PK, Sasisekharan V (1971) Studies on the conformation of amino acids. V. Conformation of amino acids with γ-atoms. Int J Pept. Protein Res 3:9

Popovic WJ, Brown JE, Adamson JW (1977) The influences of thyroid hormones on in vitro erythropoeisis: mediation by a receptor with beta adrenergic properties. J Clin Invest 60: 907

Portnay GI, O'Brian JT, Bush J, Vagenakis AG, Azizi F, Arky RA, Ingbar SH, Braverman LE (1974) The effect of starvation on the concentration and binding of thyroxine and triiodothyronine in serum and on the response to TRH. J Clin Endocrinol Metab 39:191

Premchandra BN (1978) Radioimmunoassay of reverse trriodothyronine. J Clin Endocrinol Metab 47:746

Premchandra BN, Perlstein IB, Blumenthal HT Studies on obesity. II. (1970) Slow-moving thyroxine binding globulin in the sera of normal and obese subjects. J Clin Endocrinol Metab 30:752

Ramsden DB (1975) Peripheral metabolism and action of thyroid hormones. Eden Press, Montreal

Rastogi GK, Sawhney RC, Panda NC, Tripathy BB (1974) Thyroid hormone levels in adult protein calorie malnutrition. Horm Metab Res 6:528

Ratcliffe WA, Marshall JA, Ratcliffe JG (1976) The radioimmunoassay of 3,3',5'-triiodothyronine (reverse T_3) in unextracted serum. Clin Endocrinol (Oxf) 5:631

Raz A, Goodman DS (1969) The interaction of thyroxine with human plasma prealbumin and with the prealbumin-retinol-binding complex. J Biol Chem 244:3230

Refetoff S, Selenkow HA (1968) Familial thyroxine binding globulin deficiency in a patient with Turner's syndrome (XO). N Engl J Med 278:1081

Refetoff S, Robin NI, Fang VS (1970) Parameters of thyroid function in serum of 16 selected vertebrate species: a study of PBI, serum T_4, free T_4, and the pattern of T_4 and T_3 binding to serum proteins. Endocrinology 86:793

Refetoff S, Matalon R, Bigazzi M (1972) Metabolism of L-thyroxine (T_4) and L-triiodothyronine (T_3) by human fibroblasts in tissue culture: evidence of cellular binding proteins and conversion of T_4 to T_3. Endocrinology 91:934

Refetoff S, Fang VS, Marshall JS (1975) Studies on human thyroxine-binding globulin. IX. Some physical, chemical, and biological properties of radioiodinated TBG and partially desialylated TBG. J Clin Invest 56:177

Rehn L (1884) Über die Exstirpation des Kropfs bei Morbus Basedowii. Klin Wochenschr 21:163

Reichlin S, Bollinger J, Nejad I, Sullivan P (1973) Tissue thyroid hormone concentration of rat and man determined by radioimmunoassay: biologic significance. Mt Sinai J Med (NY) 40:502

Reverdin JL, Reverdin A (1883) Note sur vingtdeux operations de goitre. Rev Med Suisse Romande 3:169

Robbins J (1975) Structure and function of thyroxine-transport proteins. In: Harland WA, Orr JS (eds) Thyroid hormone metabolism. Academic Press, New York, pp 1–22

Robbins J, Rall JE (1952) Zone electrophoresis in filter paper of serum I^{131} after radioiodide administration. Proc Soc Exp Biol Med 81:530

Robbins J, Rall JE (1957) The interaction of thyroid hormones and protein in biological fluids. Recent Progr Horm Res 13:161

Robbins J, Rall JE, Petermann ML (1957) Thyroxine binding by serum and urine proteins in nephrosis. Qualitative aspects. J Clin Invest 36:1333

Robbins J, Rall JE, Gorden P (1974) The thyroid and iodine metabolism. In: Bondy PK, Rosenberg LE (eds) Duncan's diseases of metabolism and endocrinology, 7th ed. vol 2. Saunders, Philadelphia, pp 1009–1104

Roche J, Lissitzky S, Michel R (1952a) Sur la triiodothyronine, produit intermedia re de la transformation de la diiodothyronine en thyroxine. CR Acad Sci [D] (Paris) 234:997

Roche J, Lissitzky S, Michel R (1952b) Sur la presence de triiodothyronine dans la thyroglobuline. G R Acad Sci [D] (Paris) 234:1228

Roche J, Michel R, Nunez J (1956) Sur la presence de la 3:3':5'-triiodothyronine dans le sang de rat. C R Soc Biol (Paris) 150:20

Roche J, Nunez J, Jacquemin C (1962) Nature des produits de la desidation des hormones thyroidiennes marquées simultanement par le tritium et l'iode radioactif. Biochem Biophys Acta 64:475

Rogowski P, Siersback-Nielsen K, Molholm Hansen J (1978) Urinary excretion of thyroxine and triiodothyronine in different thyroid function states in man. Acta Endocrinol (Copenh) 87: 525

Rubenstein HA, Butler VP jr, Werner SC (1973) Progressive decrease in serum triiodothyronine concentrations with human aging: radioimmunoassay following extraction of serum. J Clin Endocrinol Metab 37:247

Rudolph M, Sakurada T, Fang SL, Vagenakis AG, Braverman LE, Ingbar SH (1978) Appearance of labeled metabolites in the serum of man after the administration of labeled thyroxine, triiodothyronine (T_3), and reverse triiodothyronine (rT_3). J Clin Endocrinol Metab 36:923

Saberi M, Sterling FH, Utiger RD (1975) Reduction in extrathyroidal triiodothyronine production by propylthiouracil in man. J Clin Invest 55:218

Samuels HH, Tsai JS (1974) Thyroid hormone action, demonstration of similar receptors in isolated nuclei of rat liver and cultured GH_1 cells. J Clin Invest 53:656

Samuels HH, Stanley F, Shapiro LE (1977) Modulation of thyroid nuclear receptor levels by 3,5,3'-triiodo-L-thyronine in GH_1 cells. J Biol Chem 252:6052

Schally AV, Bowers CY, Redding TW, Barrett JF (1966) Isolation of thyrotropin releasing factor (TRF) from porcine hypothalamus. Biochem Biophys Res Commun 25:165

Schally AV, Redding TW, Bowers CY, Barrett JF (1969) Isolation and properties of porcine thyrotropin releasing hormone. J Biol Chem 244:4077

Schussler GC (1972) Thyroxine-binding globulin: specificity for the hormonally active conformation of triiodothyronine. Science 178:172

Schwartz HL, Surks MI, Oppenheimer JH (1971) Quantitation of extrathyroidal conversion of L-thyroxine to 3,5,3'-triiodo-L-thyronine in the rat. J Clin Invest 50:1124

Seal US, Doe RP (1965) Purification, some properties and composition of the corticosteroid– and thyroxine-binding globulins from human serum. Excerpta Med Intern Congr Ser 83:325

Segall-Blank M (1978) The role of defective enzyme activity in the deficient generation of triiodothyronine (T_3) from thyroxine (T_4) in fetal rabbit liver. Annu Meet Amer Thyroid Assoc., p. T-7.

Shakespear, RA, Burke CW (1976) Triiodothyronine and thyroxine in urine. I. Measurement and application. J Clin Endocrinol Metab 42:494

Shambaugh GE III (1978) Chemistry and actions of thyroid hormones: iologic and cellular effects. In: Werner SC, Ingbar SH (eds) The thyroid. Harper & Row, New York, p 115

Shenkman L, Hollander CS (1975) Measurement of the effective thyroxine ratio (ETR) in the neonate, infant and child. J Nucl Med 16:955

Silva JE, Larsen PR (1977) Pituitary nuclear 3,5,3'-triiodothyronine and thyrotropin secretion: an explanation for the effect of thyroxine. Science 198:617

Silva JE, Dick TE, Larsen PR (1978) The contribution of local tissue thyroxine monodeiodination to the nuclear 3,5,3'-triiodothyronine in pituitary, liver and kidney of euthyroid rats. Endocrinology 103:1196

Sims EAH (1976) Experimental obesity, dietary – induced thermogenesis and their clinical implications. Clin Endocrinol Metab 5:377

Singh SP, Carter AC, Kydd DM, Constanzo RR (1976) Interaction between thyroid hormones and erythrocyte membranes: competitive inhibition of binding ^{131}I-L-triiodothyronine and ^{131}I-L-thyroxine by their analogs. Endocr Res Commun 3:119

Smallridge RC, Wartofsky L, Desjardins RE, Burman KD (1978) Metabolic clearance and production rates of 3,3',5-triiodothyronine in hyperthyroid, euthyroid and hypothyroid subjects. J Clin Endocrinol Metab 47:345

Smith PE, Smith IP (1922) The repair and activation of the thyroid in the hypophysectomized tadpole by the parental administration of fresh anterior lobe of bovine hypophysis. J Med Res 43:267

Smith SJ, Bos G, Gerbrandy J, Docter R, Visser TJ, Henneman G (1978) Lowering of serum 3,3',5-triiodothyronine to thyroxine ratio in patients with myocardial infarction; relationship with extent of tissue injury. Eur J Clin Invest 8:99

Snyder SM, Cavalieri RR, Goldfine ID, Ingbar SH, Jorgensen EC (1976) Binding of thyroid hormones and their analogues to thyroxine-binding globulin in human serum. J Biol Chem 251:6489

Socolow EL, Woeber KA, Purdy RH, Holloway MT, Ingbar SH (1965) Preparation of I^{131}-labeled human serum prealbumin and its metabolism in normal and sick patients. J Clin Invest 44:1600

Solomon SS (1972) Phosphodiesterase activity of rat and human adipose tissue. J Lab Clin Med 79:598

Sorimachi K, Robbins J (1977) Metabolism of thyroid hormones by monkey hepatocarcinoma cells. J Biol Chem 252:4458

Spaulding SW, Chopra IJ, Sherwin RS, Lyall SS (1976) Effect of caloric restriction and dietary composition on serum T_3 and reverse T_3 in man. J Clin Endocrinol Metab 42:197

Spindler BJ, MacLeod KM, Ring J, Baxter JD (1975) Thyroid hormone receptors. Binding characteristics and lack of hormonal dependency for nuclear localization. J Biol Chem 250:4113

Stasilli NR, Kroc RL, Meltzer R (1959) Antigoiterogenic and calorigenic activities of thyroxine analogues in rats. Endocrinology 64:62

Sterling K (1970) The significance of circulating triiodothyronine. Recent Progr Horm Res 26:249
Sterling K (1979) Thyroid hormone action at the cell level. N Engl J Med 300:117
Sterling K, Milch PO (1974) Thermal inactivation of thyroxine binding globulin for direct radioimmunoassay of triiodothyronine. J Clin Endocrinol Metab 38:866
Sterling K, Milch PO (1975) Thyroid hormone binding by a component of mitochondrial membrane. Proc Natl Asad Sci USA 72:3275
Sterling K, Lashof JC, Man EB (1954) Disappearance from serum of I^{131}-labeled L-thyroxine and L-triiodothyronine in euthyroid subjects. J Clin Invest 33:1031
Sterling K, Bellabarba D, Newman ES, Brenner M (1969) Determination of triiodothyronine concentration in human serum. J Clin Invest 48:1150
Sterling K, Refetoff S, Selenkow HA (1970 a) T_3 thyrotoxicosis due to elevated serum triiodothyronine levels. JAMA 213:571
Sterling K, Brenner MA, Newman ES (1970 b) Conversion of thyroxine to triiodothyronine in normal human subjects. Science 169:1099
Sterling K, Hamada S, Takemura Y, Brenner MA, Newman ES, Inada M (1971) Preparation and properties of thyroxine binding alpha globulin (TBG). J Clin Invest 50:1758
Sterling K, Brenner M, Saldhana VF (1972) Conversion of thyroxine to triiodothyronine by cultured human cells. Science 179:1000
Sterling K, Milch PO, Brenner MA, Lazarus JH (1977) Thyroid hormone action: the mitochondrial pathway. Science 197:996
Sterling K, Lazarus JH, Milch PO, Sakurada T, Brenner MA (1978) Mitochondrial thyroid hormone receptor: localization and physiological significance. Science, 201, 1126
Suda A, Chambers J jr. Thurston C, Pittman C (1977) Thyroid hormone kinetics in the fasting and diabetic subjects. Clin Res 25:516
Suda AK, Pittman CS, Chambers JB, Ray GY (1978 a) The etiology of the "low T_3 syndrome" and dietary therapy. Ann Meet Endocr Soc p 112
Suda AK, Pittman CS, Shimizu T, Chambers JB, jr (1978 b) The production and metabolism of 3,5,3'-triiodothyronine and 3,3',5'-triiodothyronine in normal and fasting subjects. J Clin Endocrinol Metab 47:1311
Sullivan PRC, Bollinger JA, Reichlin S (1973) Selective deficiency of tissue triiodothyronine: a proposed mechanism of elevated free thyroxine in the euthyroid sick. J Clin Invest 52:83 a
Surks MI, Oppenheimer JH (1964) Postoperative changes in the concentration of thyroxine binding prealbumin and serum free thyroxine. J Clin Endocrinol Metab 24:794
Surks MI, Oppenheimer JH (1969) Formation of iodoprotein during the peripheral metabolism of 3,5,3'-triiodo-L-thyronine-^{125}I in euthyroid man and rat. J Clin Invest 48:685
Surks MI, Oppenheimer JH (1971) Metabolism of phenolic- and tyrosyl-ring labeled L-thyroxine in human beings and rats. J Clin Endocrinol Metab 33:612
Surks MI, Oppenheimer JH (1976) Isolation and characterization of thyroid hormone receptors. In: Levey GS (ed) Hormone-receptor interaction. Dekker, New York, pp 373
Surks MI, Schadlow AR, Oppenheimer JH (1972) A new radioimmunoassay for plasma L-triiodothyronine: measurements in thyroid disease and in patients maintained on hormone replacement. J Clin Invest 51:3104
Surks MI, Schadlow AR, Stock JM, Oppenheimer JH (1973 a) Determination of iodothyronine absorption and conversion of L-thyroxine (T_4) to L-triiodothyronine (T_3) using turnover rate techniques. J Clin Invest 52:805
Surks MI, Koerner D, Dillman W, Oppenheimer JH (1973 b) Limited capacity binding sites for L-triiodothyronine in rat liver nuclei. J Biol Chem 248, 7066 (1973 b)
Tabachnik M, Korcek L (1978) Thyroxine binding interactions: Binding constants for interaction of thyroxine analogues with the thyroxine binding site on human thyroxine-binding globulin. Biochim Biophys Acta 537:169
Tait JF (1963) The use of isotopic steroid for the measurement of production rates in vivo. J Clin Endocrinol Metab 23:1285
Takeda Y, Reeve EB (1963) Studies of the metabolism and distribution of albumin with autologous I^{131}-albumin in healthy men. J Lab Clin Med 61:18
Tata JR (1969) The action of thyroid hormones. Gen Comp Endocrinol [Suppl] 2:385
Tata JF, Shellabarger CJ (1959) An explanation for the difference between mammals and birds in their response to thyroxine and triiodothyronine. Biochem J 71:3P
Taurog A, Chaikoff IL (1948) The nature of circulating thyroid hormone. J Biol Chem 176:639

Thorson SC, McIntosh HW, Willms M (1969) Triiodothyronine binding affinity for thyroxine binding globulin in serum form normal subjects and from hyperthyroid, hypothyroid and pregnant patients. Acta Endocrinol (Copenh) 62:555

Tomich EG, Woollett EA, Pratt MA (1960) Some biological actions of iodo-L-thyronines. J Endocrinol 20:65

Tomita K, Lardy HA, Larson EC, Albright EC (1957) Enzymatic conversion of thyroxine to tetraiodothyroacetic acid and of triiodothyronine to triiodothyroacetic acid. J Biol Chem 224:387

Torresani J, Anselmet A, Wahl R (1978) Properties of solubilized nuclear triiodothyronine binding proteins. Mol Cell Endocrinol 9:321

Uller RP, van Herle AJ, Chopra IJ (1973) Comparison of alterations in circulating thyroglobulin, triiodothyronine and thyroxine in response to exogenous (bovine) and endogenous (human) thyrotropin. J Clin Endocrinol Metab 37:741

Vagenakis AG, Burger A, Portnay GI, Rudolph M, O'Brian JT, Azizi F, Arky RA, Nicod P, Ingbar SH, Braverman LE (1975) Diversion of peripheral thyroxine metabolism from activating to inactivating pathways during complete fasting. J Clin Endocrinol Metab 41:191

Vagenakis AG, Portnay GI, O'Brian JT, Rudolph M, Arky RA, Ingbar SH, Braverman LE (1977) Effect of starvation on the production and metabolism of thyroxine and triiodothyronine in euthyroid obese patients. J Clin Endocrinol Metab 45:1305

Van der Heijden SPN, Griffith EAH, Chandler WD, Robertson BE (1975) Conformations of bridged diphenyls. VII. Crystal structure of 2-(4-carbomethoxy-2′-nitrophenoxy)-1,3,5-trimethylbenzene. Can J Chem 53:2084

Van Lenten L, Ashwell G (1972) The binding of desialylated glycoproteins by plasma membranes of rat liver: development of a quantiatative inhibition assay. J Biol Chem 247:4633

Van Middlesworth L (1974) Handbook of physiology, Section 7: Endocrinology, vol III, Metabolism and excretion of thyroid hormones. In: Solomon DH, Greer MA (eds) Thyroid. American Physiological Society, Washington DC p 215

Verhoeven RP, Visser TJ, Docter R, Henneman G, Schalekamp MADH (1977) Plasma thyroxine, 3,3′,5′-triiodothyronine during B-adrenergic blockade in hyperthyroidism. J Clin Endocrinol Metab 44:1002

Vignati L, Finley RJ, Haag S, Aski TT (1978) Protein conservation during prolonged fast: a function of triiodothyronine (T_3) levels. Clin Res 26:563A

Vinik AI, Kalk WJ, McLaren H, Hendricks S, Primstone BL (1975) Fasting blunts the TSH response to synthetic thyrotropin releasing hormone (TRH). J Clin Endocrinol Metab 40:509

Visser TJ, van der Does-Tobe I, Docter R, Henneman G (1975) Conversion of thyroxine into triiodothyronine by rat liver homogenate. Biochem J 150:489

Visser TJ, Does-Tove IVD, Docter R, Henneman G (1976) Conversion of thyroxine into triiodothyronine by rat liver homogenate. In: Robbins J, Braverman LE (eds) Thyroid research. Excerpta Medica, Amsterdam, p 235

Visser TJ, Lamberts SWJ, Wilson JHP, Docter R, Henneman G (1978 a) Serum thyroid hormone concentrations during prolonged reduction of dietary intake. Metabolism 27:405

Visser TJ, Fekkes D, Docter R, Henneman G (1978 b) Sequential deiodination of thyroxine in rat liver homogenates. Biochem J 174: 221

Volpert EM, Grinberg R, Werner SC (1962) Studies with mouse pituitary thyrotropic tumors. IV. Presence of 3,5,3′-triiodothyronine in certain mouse pituitary tumors after injection of labeled L-thyroxine. Endocrinology 71:361

Wallack MS, Adelberg HH, Nicoloff JT (1970) Thyroid suppression test using single dose of I-thyroxine. N Engl J Med 283: 402

Wartofsky L, Burman KD, Dimond RC, Earll JM (1977) Studies on the nature of thyroidal suppression during acute falciparum malaria: integrity of pituitary response to TRH and alterations in serum T_3 and reverse T_3. J Clin Endocrinol Metab 44:85

Weeke J, Orskov H (1973) Synthesis of ^{125}I-monolabelled 3,5,3′-triiodothyronine and thyroxine of maximum specific activity for radioimmunoassay. Scand J Clin Lab Invest 32:357

Weeks CM, Cody V, Pokrywiecki S, Rohrer DC, Duax WL (1974) Applications of the PROPHET System in correlating crystallographic structural data with biological information. AFIPS Conf Proc 43:469

Werner SC, Spooner M (1955) A new and simple test for hyperthyroidism employing L-triiodothyronine and the 24 hours ^{131}I uptake method. Bull NY Acad Med 31:137

Westgren U, Burger A, Ingemansson S, Melander A, Tibblin S, Wahlin E (1976) Blood levels of 3,5,3'-triiodothyronine and thyroxine: differences between children, adults, and elederly subjects. Acta Med Scand 200:493

Westgren U, Melander A, Wahlen E, Lindgren J (1977 a) Divergent effects of 6-propylthiouracil on 3,5,3'-triiodothyronine (T_3) and 3,3',5'-triiodothyronine (rT_3) serum levels in man. Acta Endocrinol (Copenh) 85:345

Westgren U, Ahren B, Burger A, Ingemansson S, Melander A (1977 b) Effects of dexamethasone, desoxycorticosterone, and ACTH on serum concentrations of thyroxine, 3,5,3'-triiodothyronine and 3,3',5'-triiodothyronine. Acta Med Scand 202:89

Wharton T (1656) Adenographia: sive, glandularum totius corporis descriptio. London. Cited by Rolleston HD (1936) The endocrine organs. In: Health and Disease. Oxford University Press, London

Wiersinga WM, Touber JL (1977) The influence of B-adrenoreceptor blocking agents on plasma thyroxine and triiodothyronine. J Clin Endocrinol Metab 45:293

Williams RJP (1977) Flexible drug molecules and dynamic receptors. Angew Chem [Engl] 16:766

Winzler RJ, Notrica SR (1952) Association of thyroxine with plasma proteins. Fed Proc 11:312

Wiswell JG, Coronho V (1962) Disappearance of I^{131}-triiodothyronine from the plasma in the presence of fever. J Clin Endocrinol Metab 22:657

Woeber KA, Ingbar SH (1973) Metabolism of L-thyroxine by phagocytosing human leukocytes. J Clin Invest 52:1706

Woeber KA, Sobel RJ, Ingbar SH, Sterling K (1970) The peripheral metabolism of triiodothyronine in normal subjects and in patients with hyperthyroidism. J Clin Invest 49:643

Wolff J, Standaert ME, Rall JE (1961) Thyroxine displacement from serum proteins and depression of serum protein-bound iodine by certain drugs. J Clin Invest 40:1373

Wu SY, Chopra IJ, Nakamura Y, Solomon DH, Bennett LR (1976) A radioimmunoassay for measurement of 3,3'-L-diiodothyronine. J Clin Endocrinol Metab 43:682

Wu SY, Chopra IJ, Solomon DH, Bennett LR (1978 a) Changes in circulating iodothyronines in euthyroid and hyperthyroid subjects given ipodate (oragrafin), an agent for oral cholecystography. J Clin Endocrinol Metab 46:691

Wu SY, Chopra IJ, Solomon DH, Johnson DE (1978 b) The effect of repeated administration of ipodate (oragrafin) in hyperthyroidism. J Clin Endocrinol Metab 47:1358

Wu SY, Klein AH, Chopra IJ, Fisher DA (1978 c) Alterations in tissue thyroxine 5'-monodeiodinating activity in perinatal period. Endocrinology 103:235

Wynn J, Gibbs R (1962) Thyroxine degradation. II. Products of thyroxine degradation by rat liver microsomes. J Biol Chem 237:3499

Yamada T, Kaplowitz N, Chopra IJ (1978) Mechanism of propylthiouracil (PTU) inhibition of hepatic thyroxine 5'-monodeiodinase. Clin Res 26:660A

Zenker N, Jorgensen EC (1959) Thyroxine analogs, I. Synthesis of 3,5-Diiodo-4-(2'-alkylphenoxy)-DL-phenylalanines. J Am Chem Soc 81:4643

Subject Index

Volume 9: R. E. Mancini
Immunologic Aspects of Testicular Function
1976. 36 figures, 8 tables. IX, 114 pages
ISBN 3-540-07496-1

Volume 8: E. Gurpide
Tracer Methods in Hormone Research
1975. 35 figures. XI, 188 pages
ISBN 3-540-07039-7

Volume 7: E. W. Horton
Prostaglandins
1972. 97 figures. XI, 197 pages
ISBN 3-540-05571-1

Volume 6: K. Federlin
Immunopathology of Insulin
Clinical and Experimental Studies
1971. 53 figures. XIII, 185 pages
ISBN 3-540-05408-1

Volume 5: J. Müller
Regulation of Aldosterone Biosynthesis
1971. 19 figures. VII, 137 pages
ISBN 3-540-05213-5

Volume 4: U. Westphal
Steroid-Protein Interactions
1971. 144 figures. XIII, 567 pages
ISBN 3-540-05312-3

Volume 3: F. G. Sulman
Hypothalamic Control of Lactation
In collaboration with numerous experts.
1970. 58 figures. XII, 235 pages
ISBN 3-540-04973-8

Volume 2: K. B. Eik-Nes, E. C. Horning
Gas Phase Chromatography of Steroids
1968. 85 figures. XV, 382 pages
ISBN 3-540-04277-6

Volume 1: S. Ohno
Sex Chromosomes and Sex-linked Genes
1967. 33 figures. X, 192 pages
ISBN 3-540-03934-1

Springer-Verlag
Berlin
Heidelberg
New York

MIX
Papier aus verantwortungsvollen Quellen
Paper from responsible sources
FSC® C105338

If you have any concerns about our products,
you can contact us on
ProductSafety@springernature.com

In case Publisher is established outside the EU,
the EU authorized representative is:
Springer Nature Customer Service Center GmbH
Europaplatz 3, 69115 Heidelberg, Germany

Printed by Libri Plureos GmbH
in Hamburg, Germany